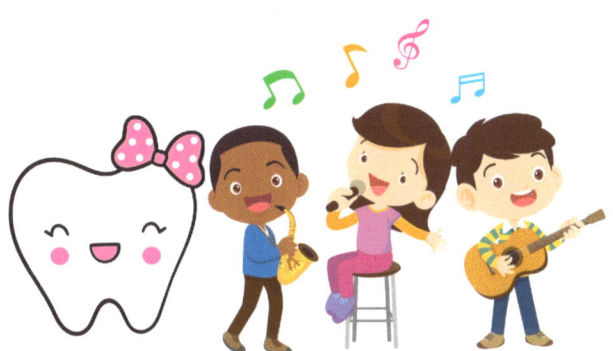

Book Learning Kids About Dental Hygiene

2-9 Y

Ryan
Go To The Dentist

By Dr A Abuzaid

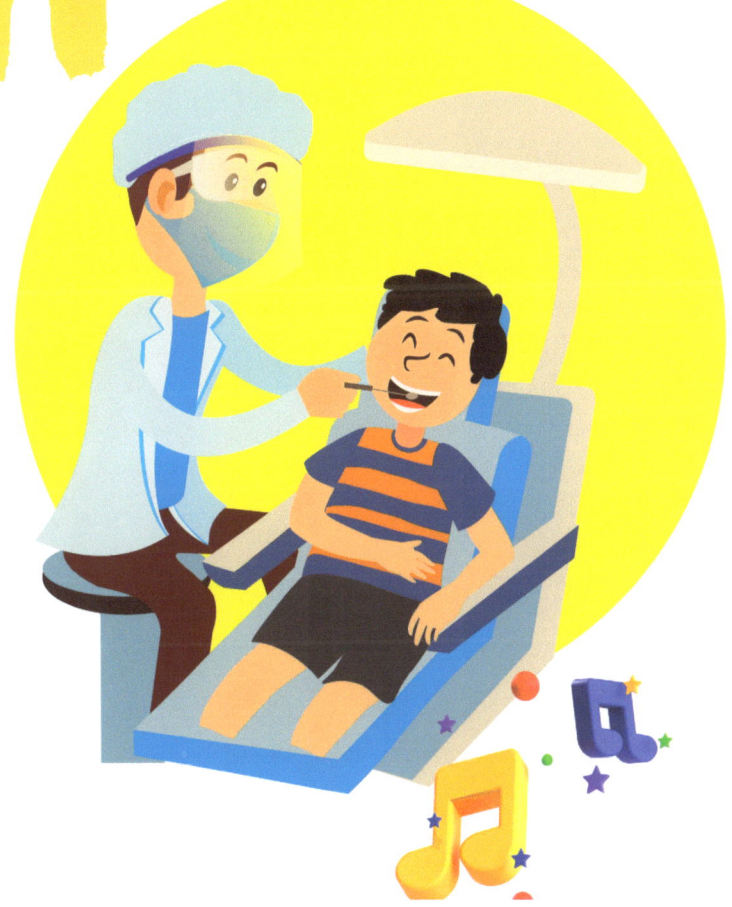

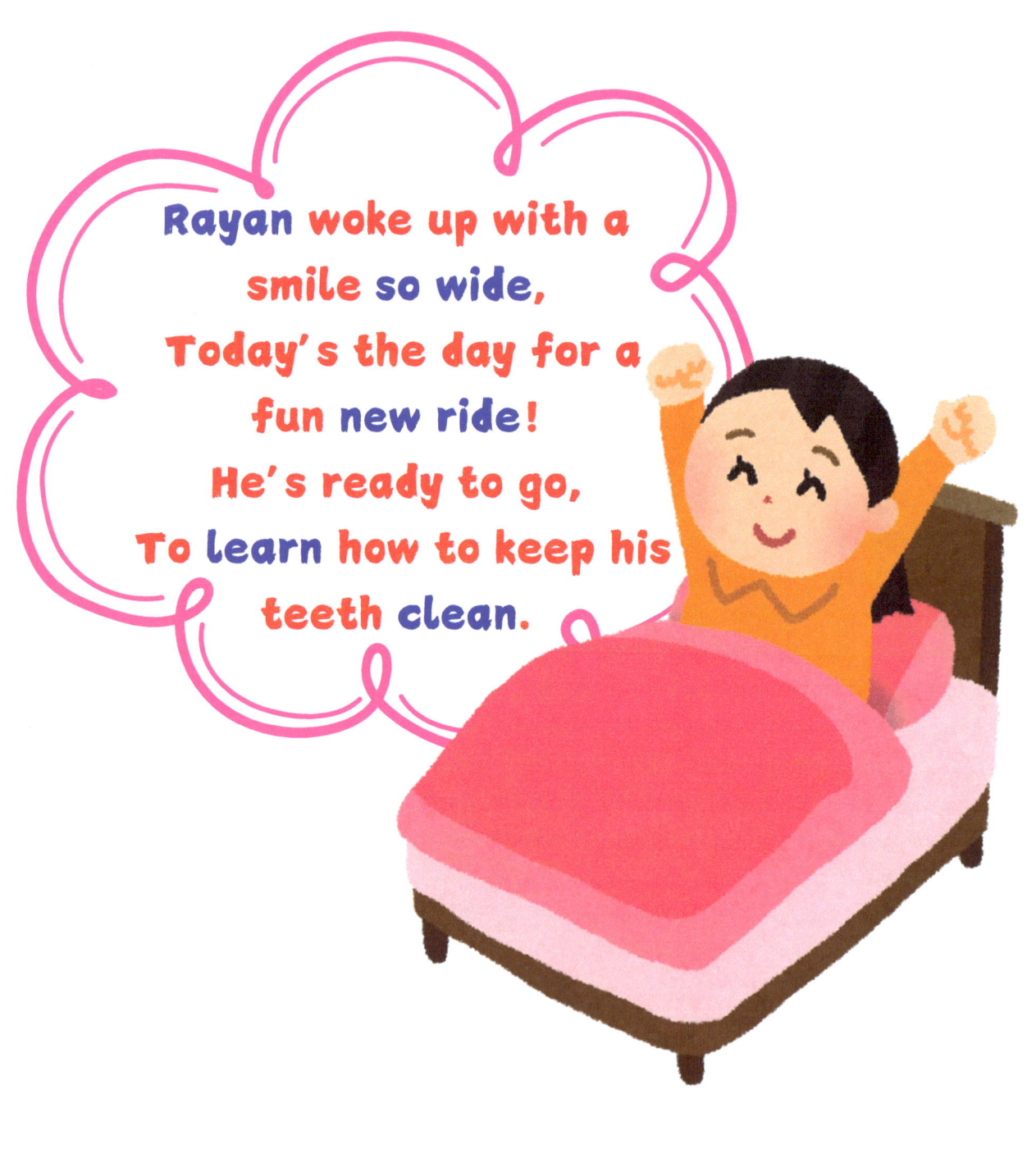

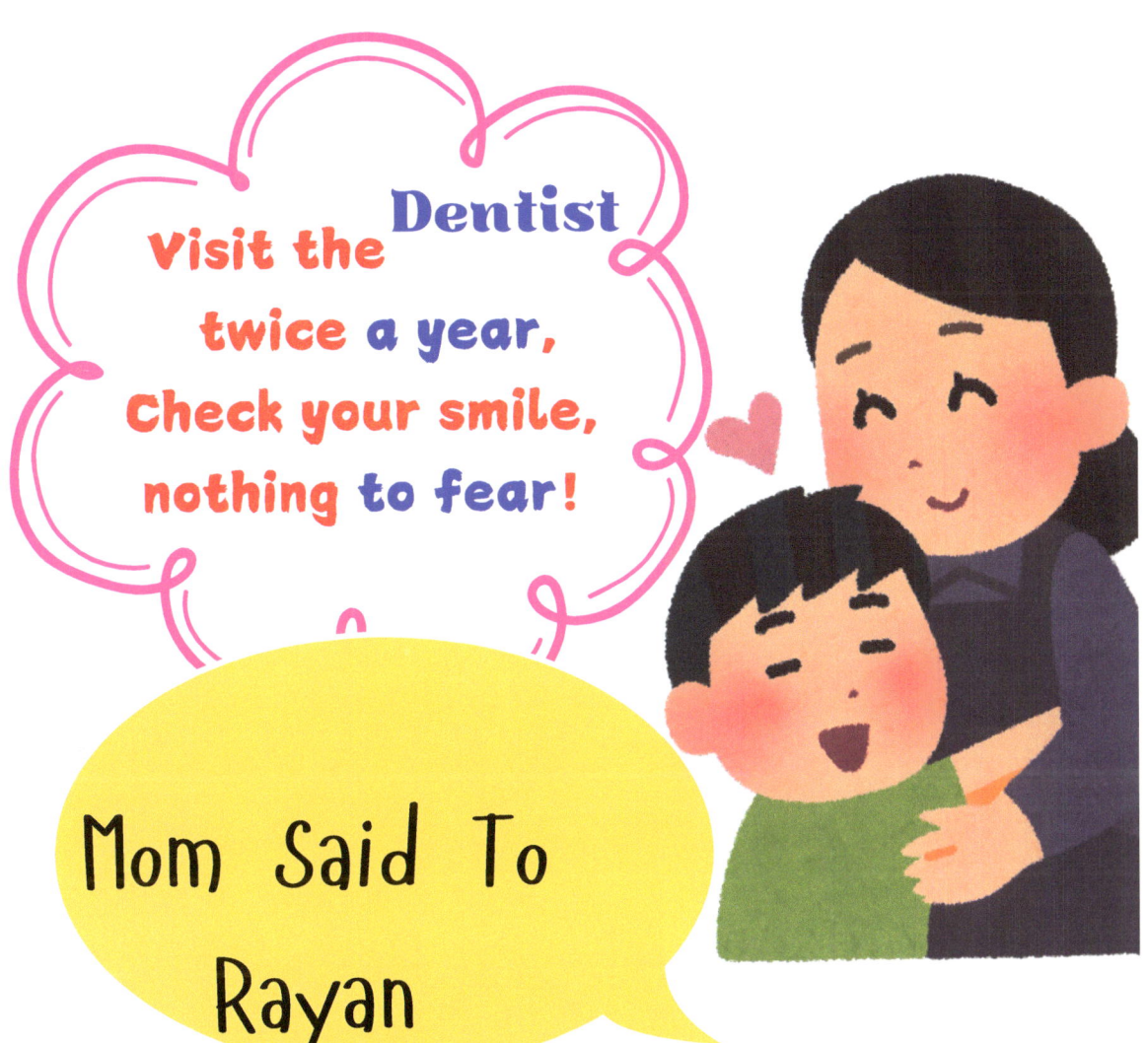

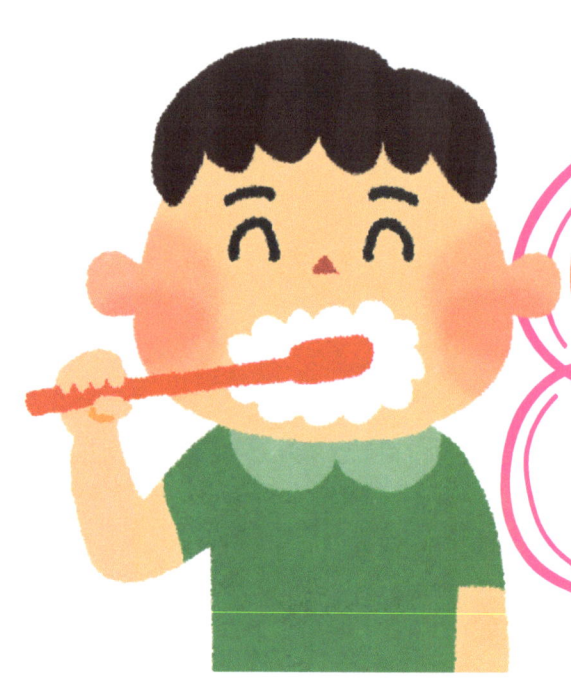

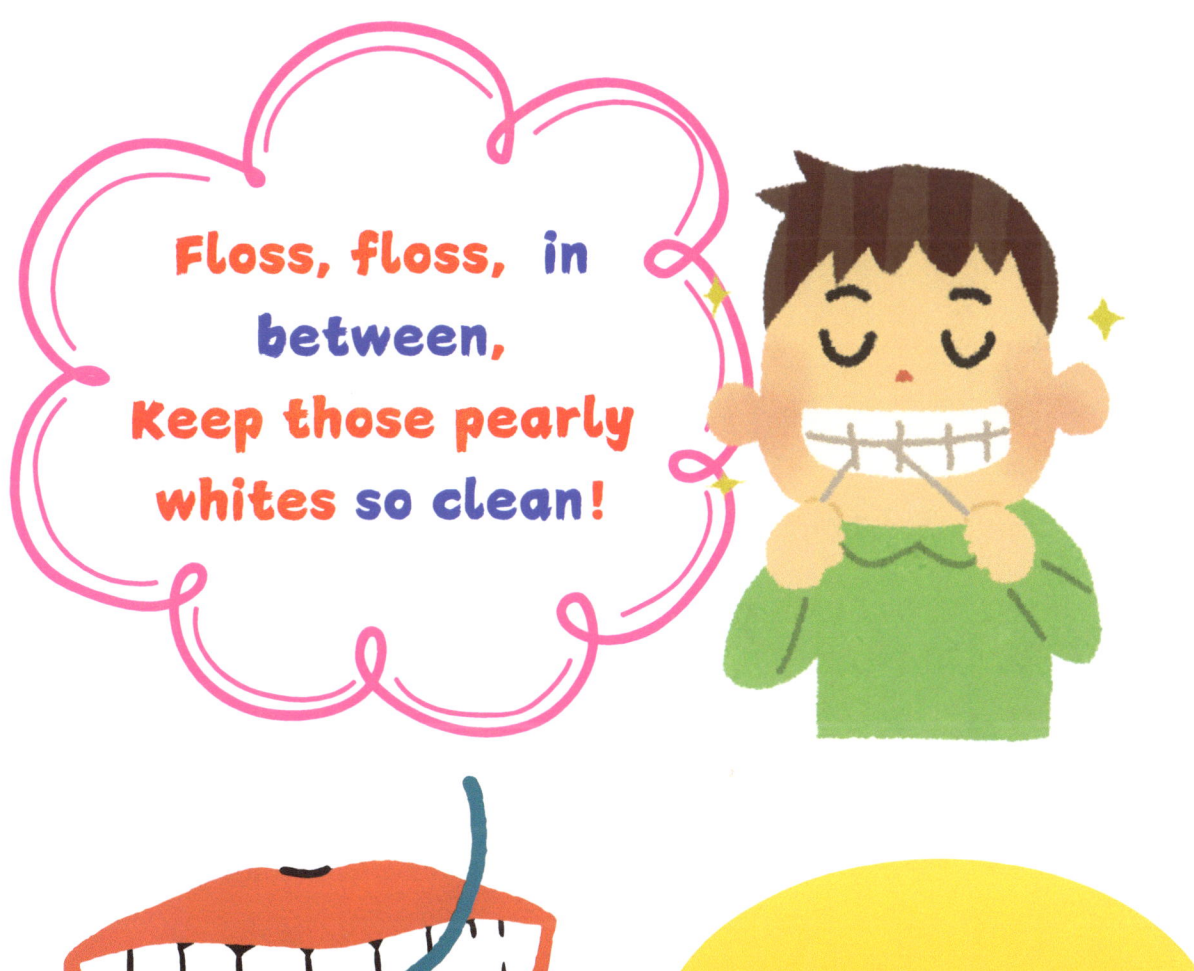

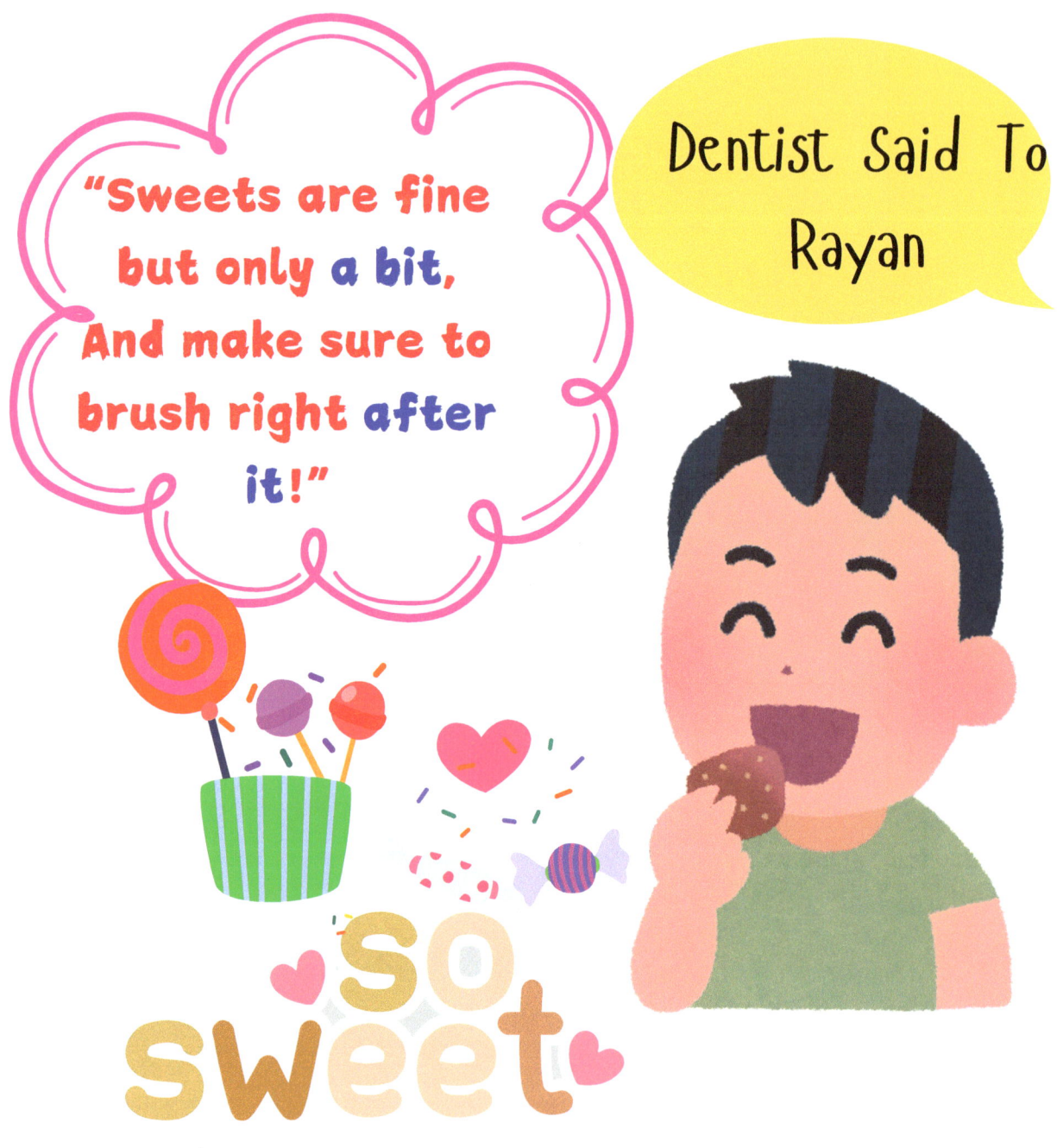

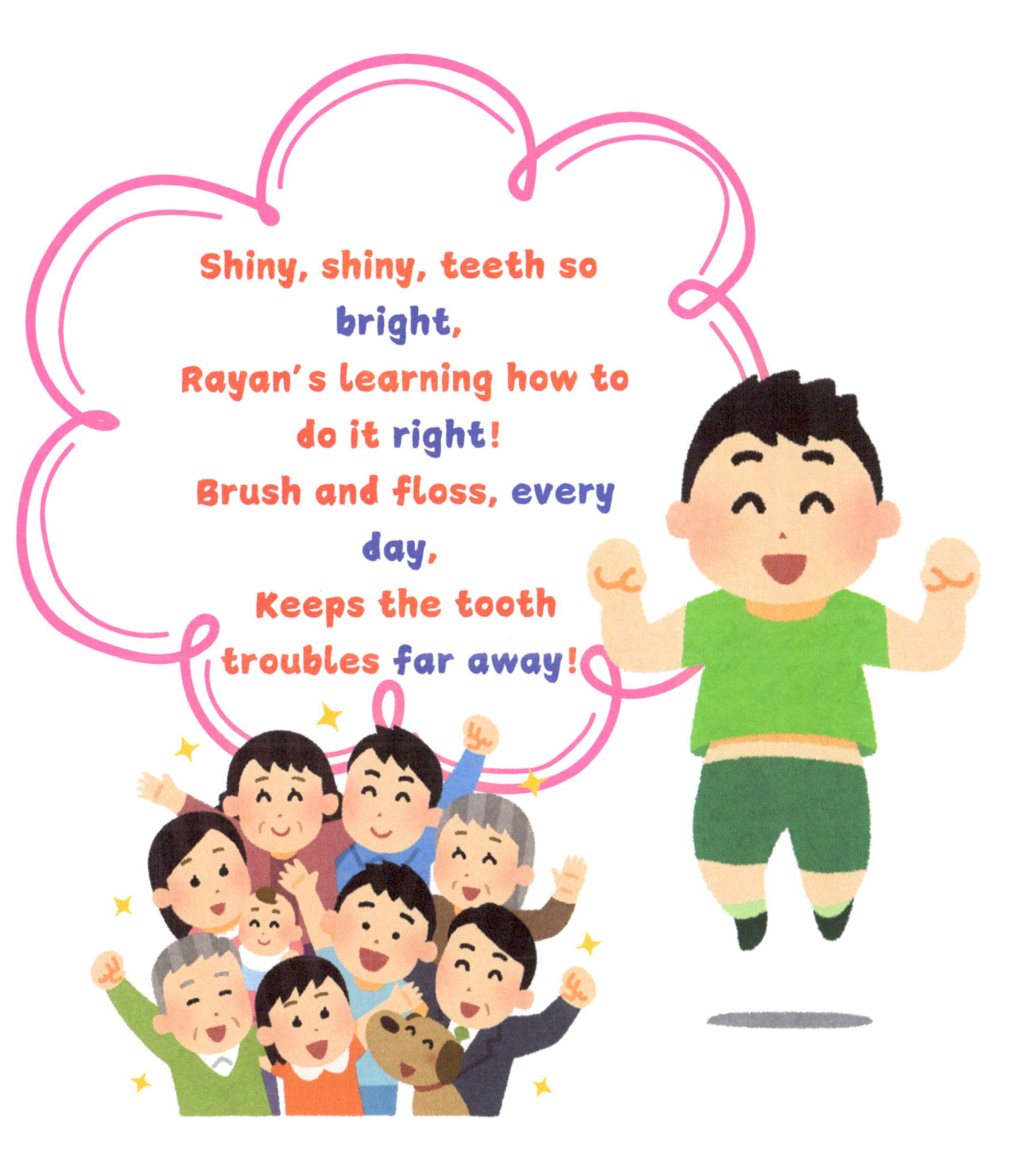

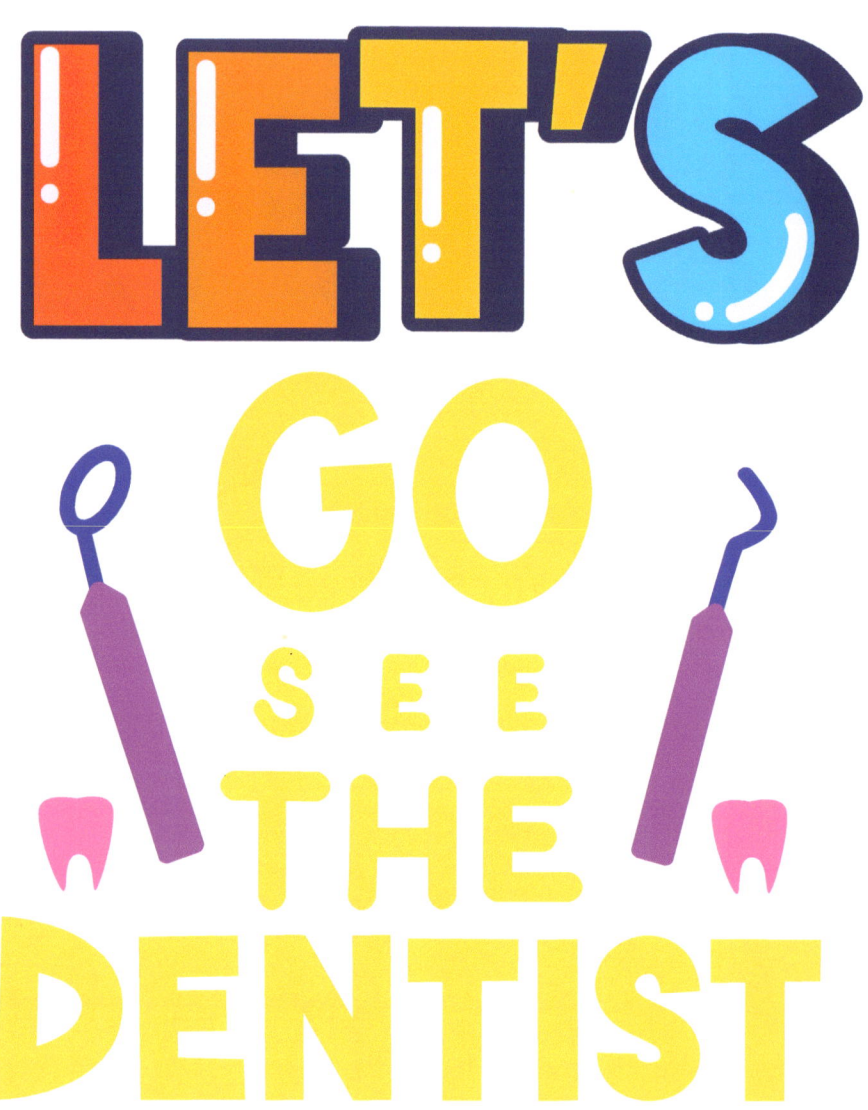

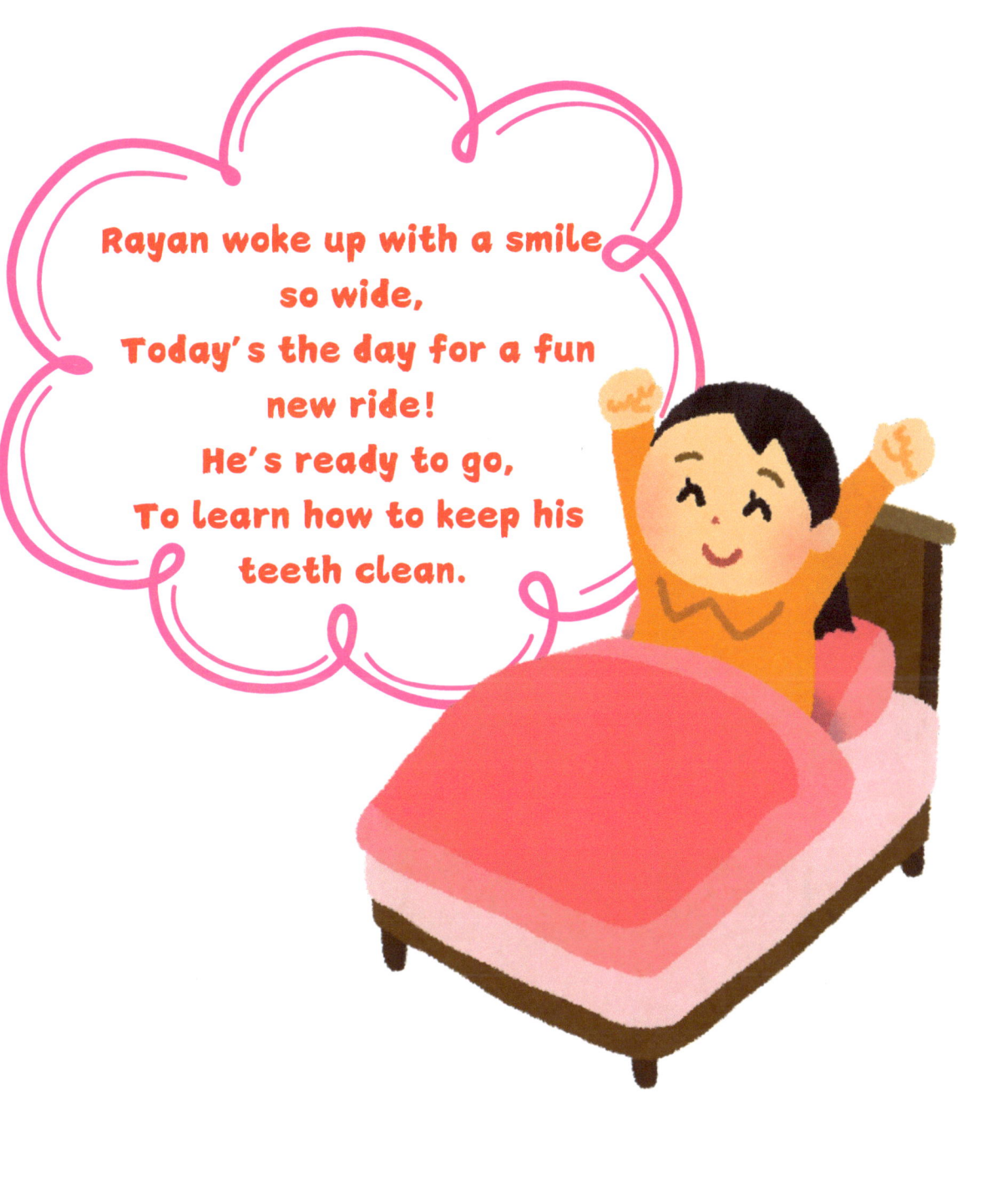

Rayan woke up with a smile so wide,
Today's the day for a fun new ride!
He's ready to go,
To learn how to keep his teeth clean.

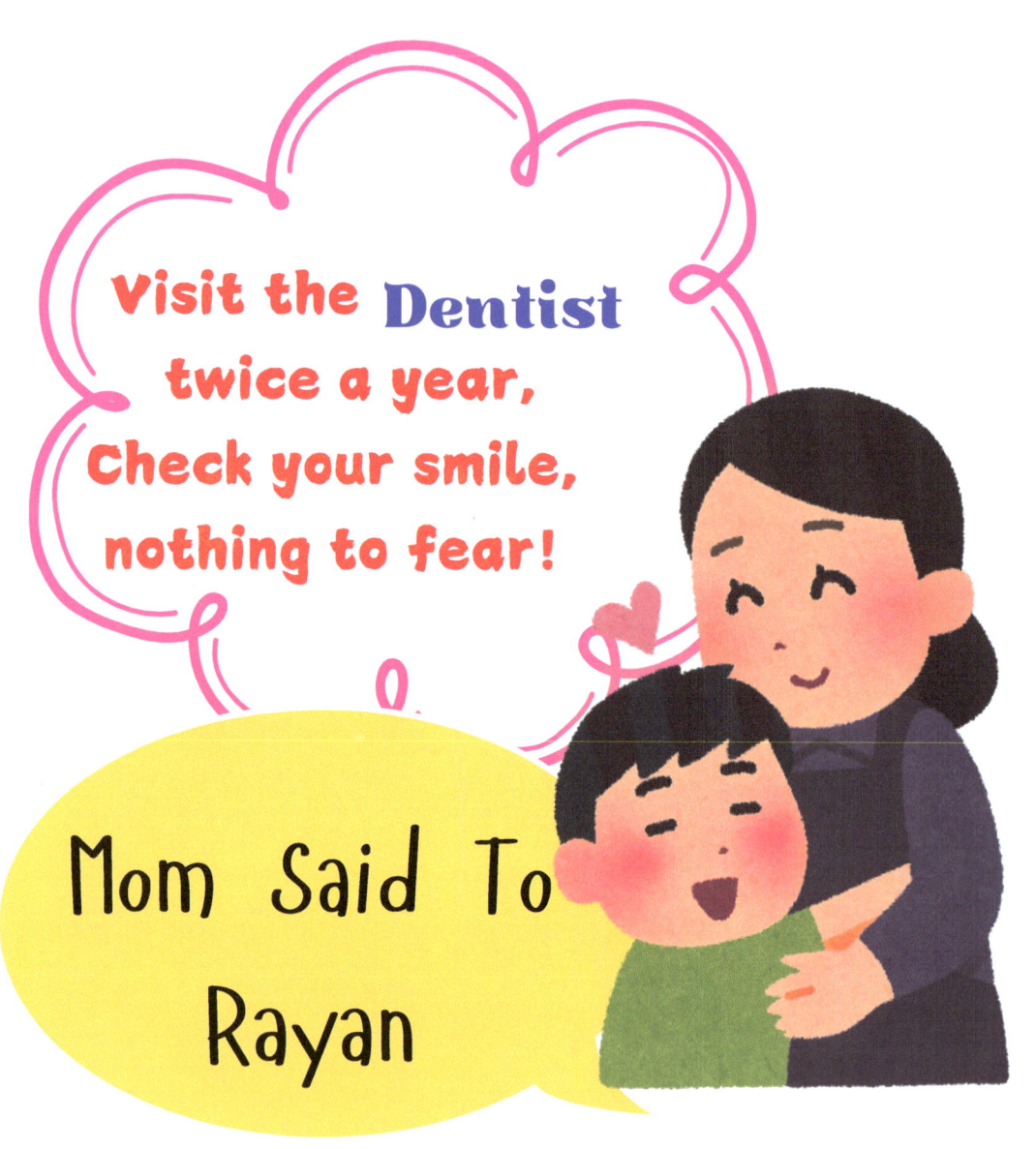

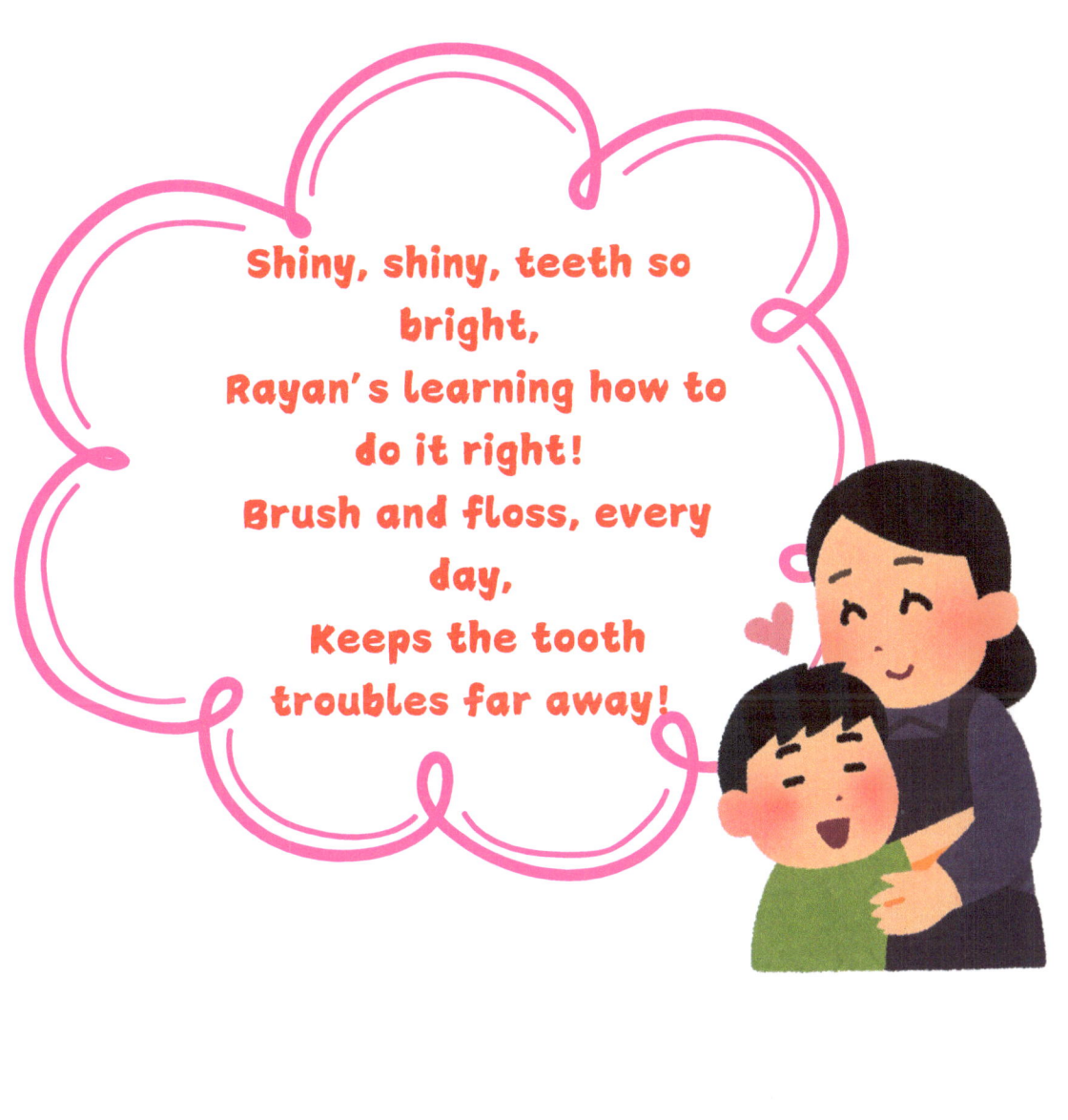

The dentist greeted Rayan with cheer,
"No need to worry, nothing to fear!
We'll check your teeth, it's quick and fun,
And then you'll see how it's all done!"

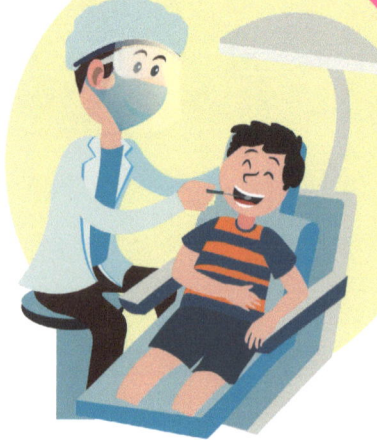

Dentist Said To Rayan

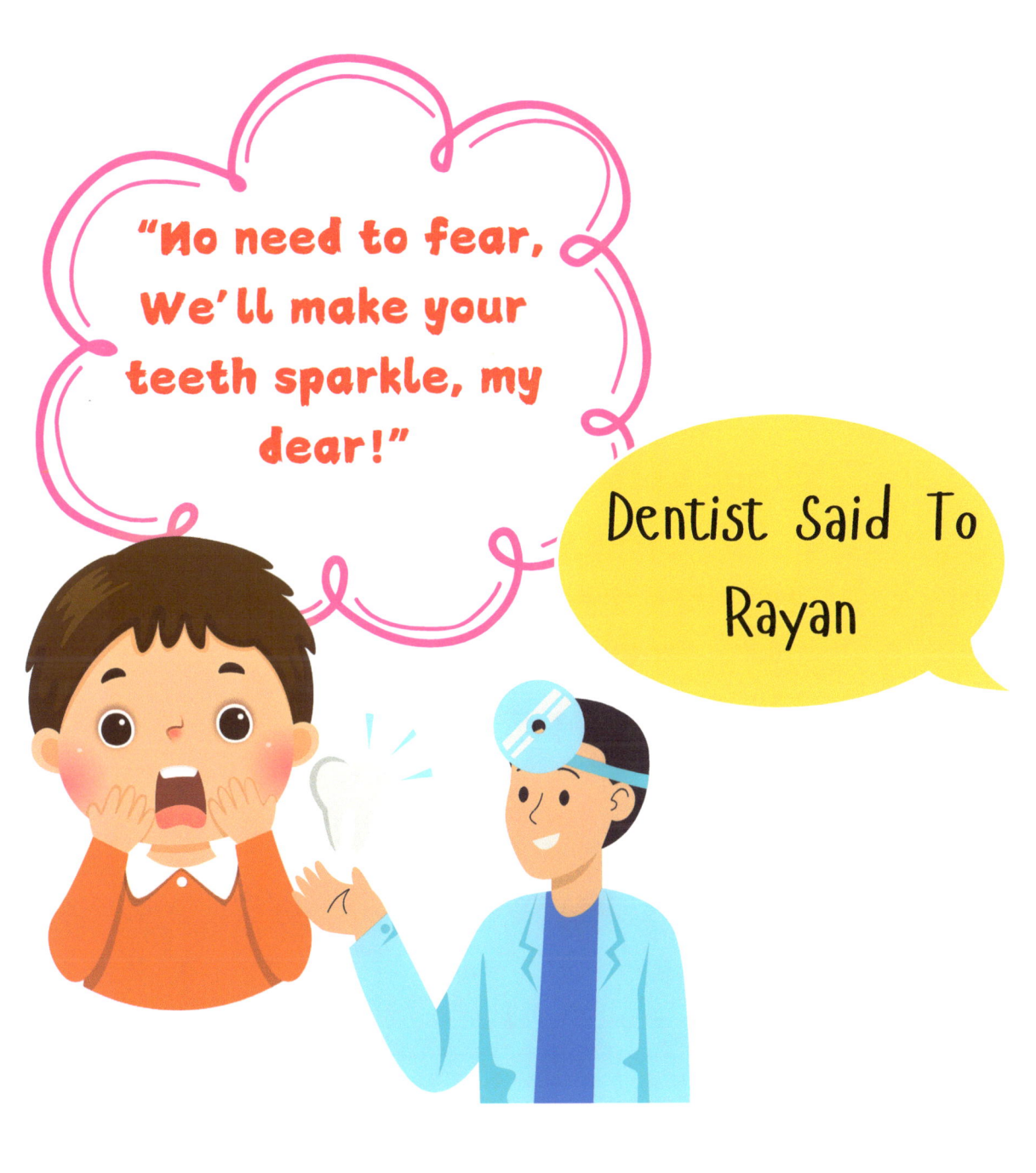

Rayan opened his mouth so wide,
The dentist looked, then smiled with pride.
"Your teeth are strong, your gums are pink,
But here's what you need to know, I think!"

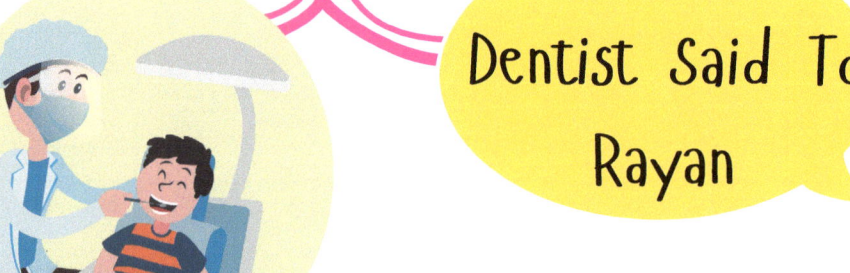

Dentist Said To Rayan

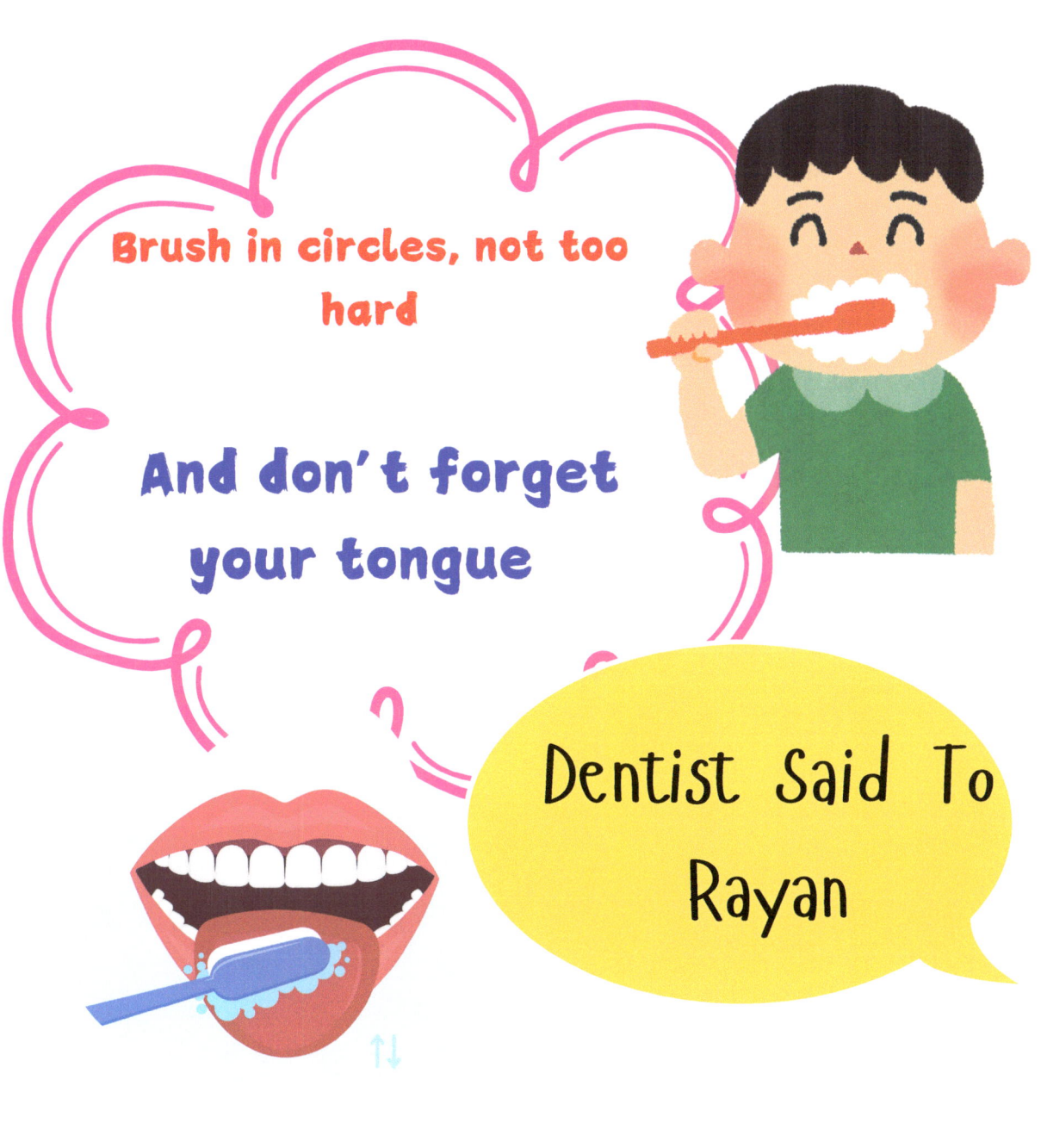

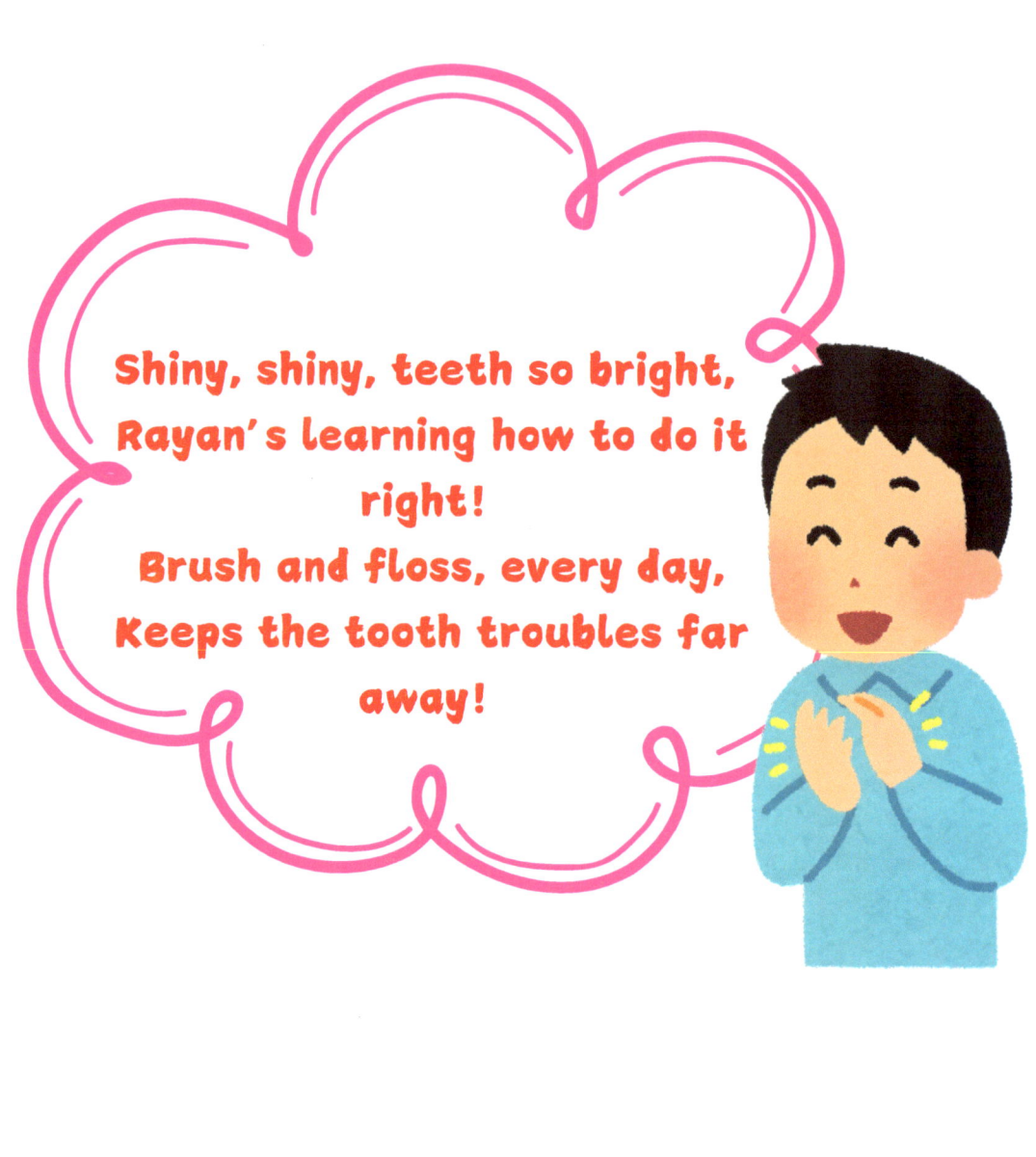

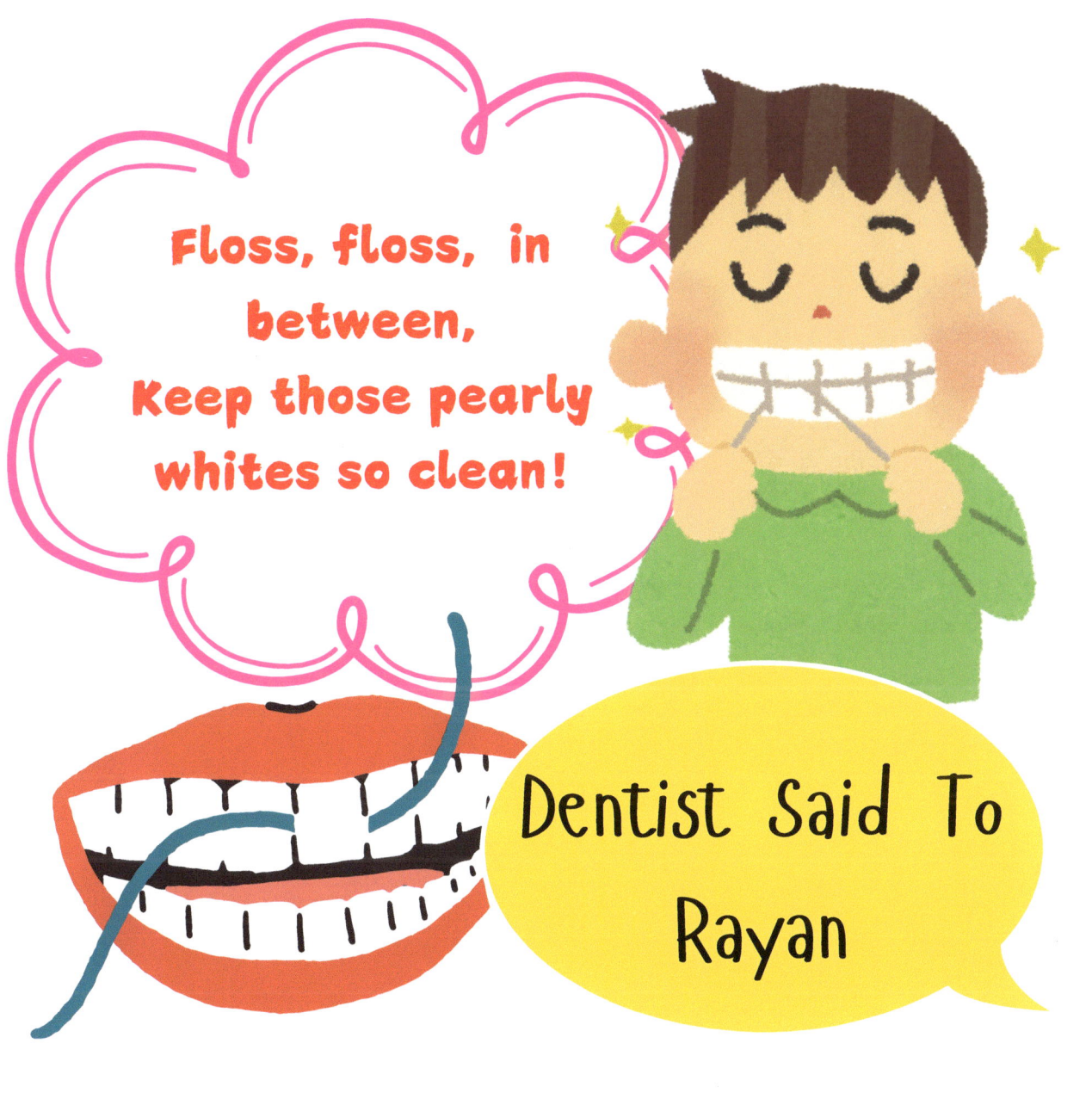

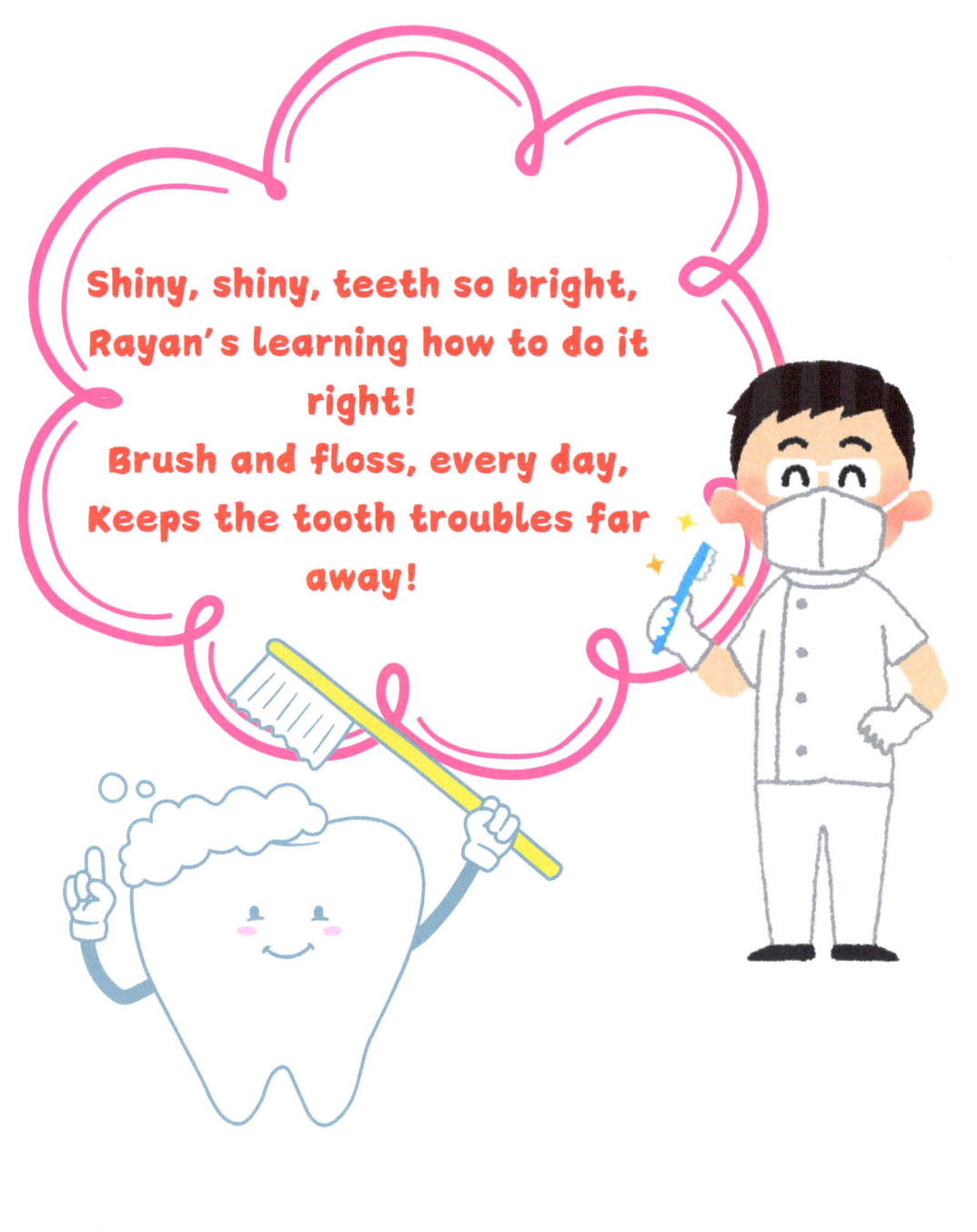

Dentist Said To Rayan

"Sweets are fine but only a bit, And make sure to brush right after it!"

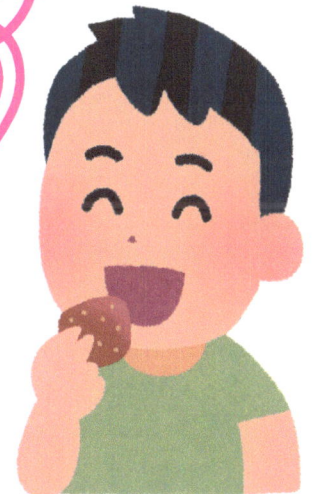

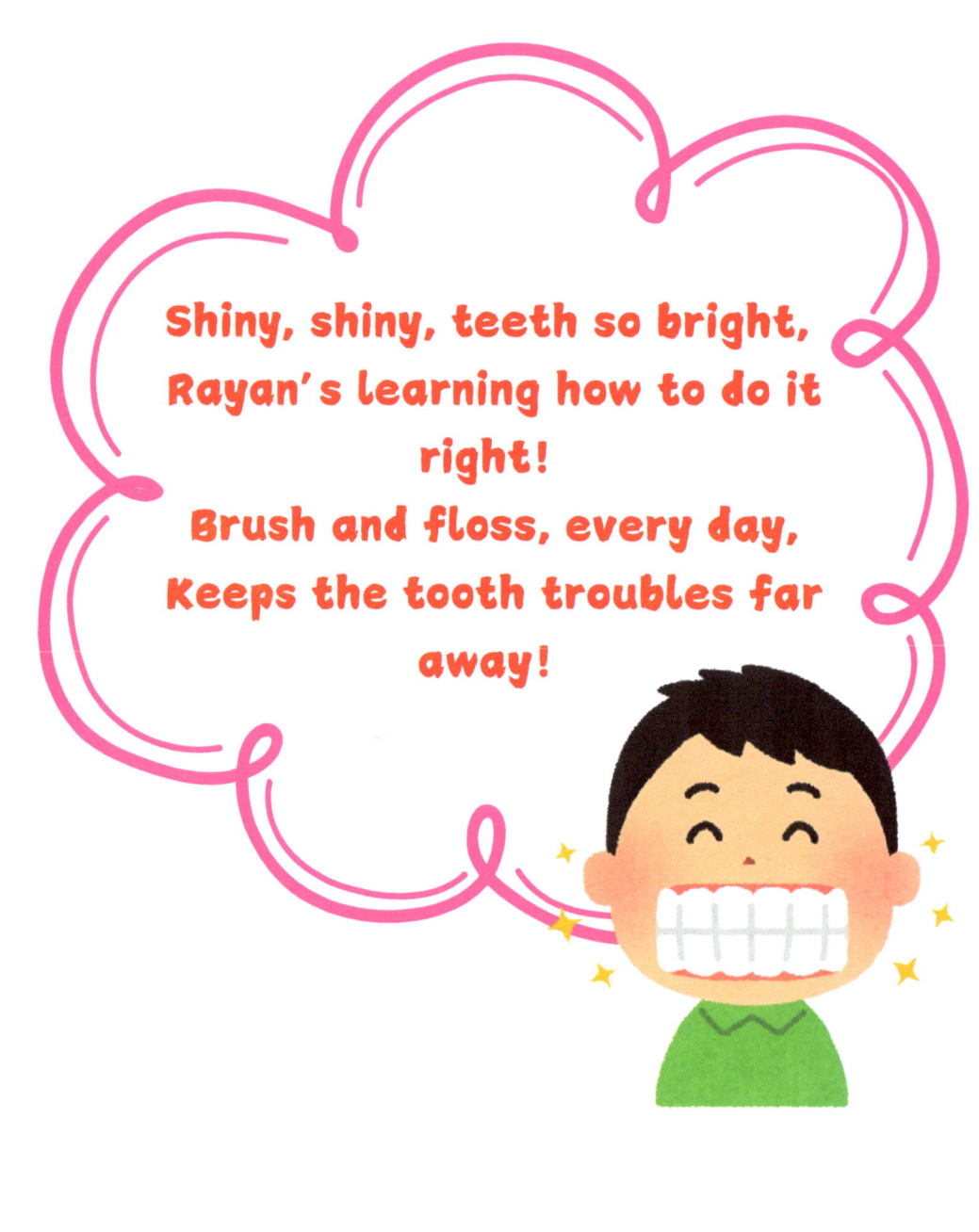

Shiny, shiny, teeth so bright,
Rayan's learning how to do it right!
Brush and floss, every day,
Keeps the tooth troubles far away!

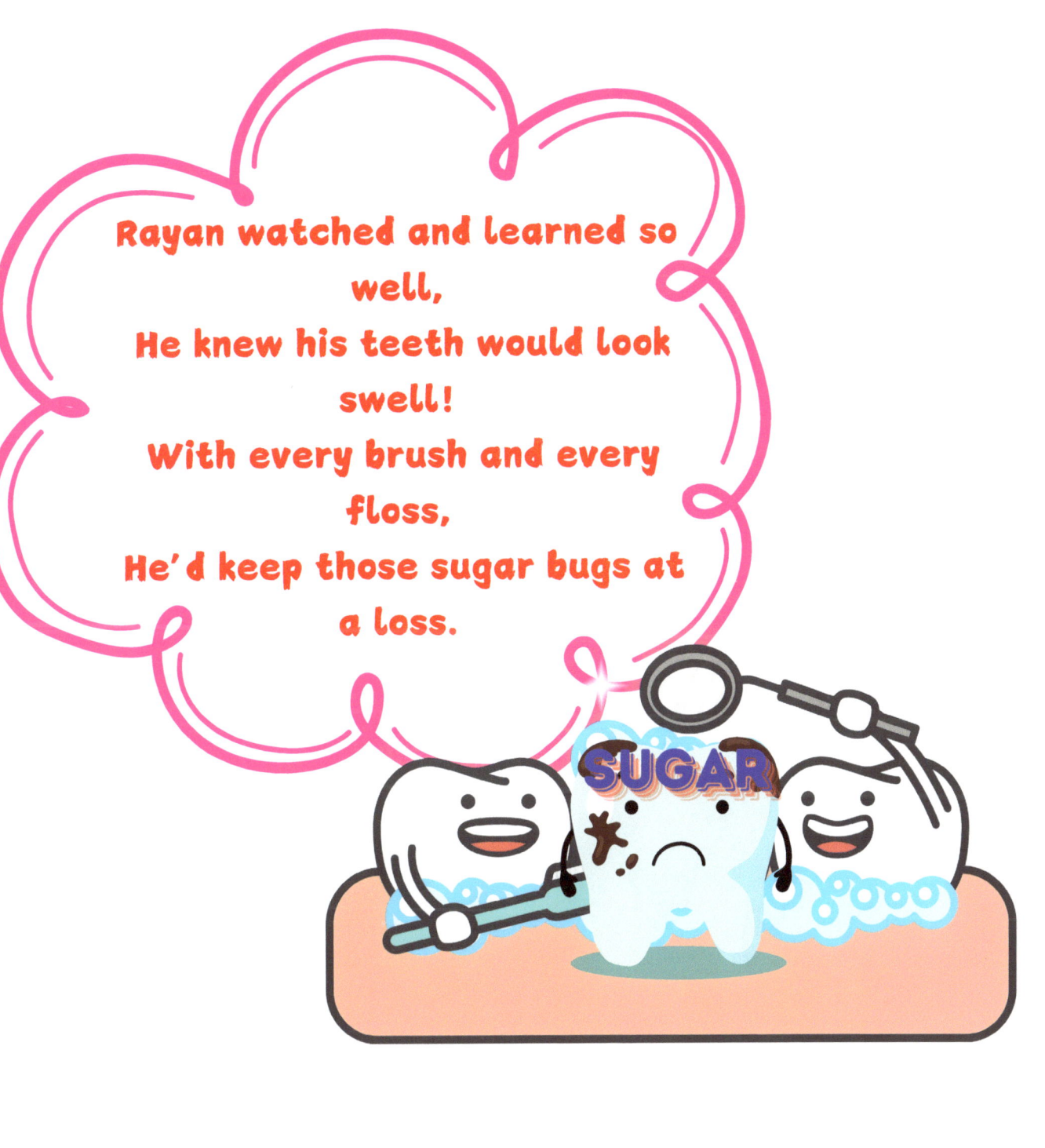

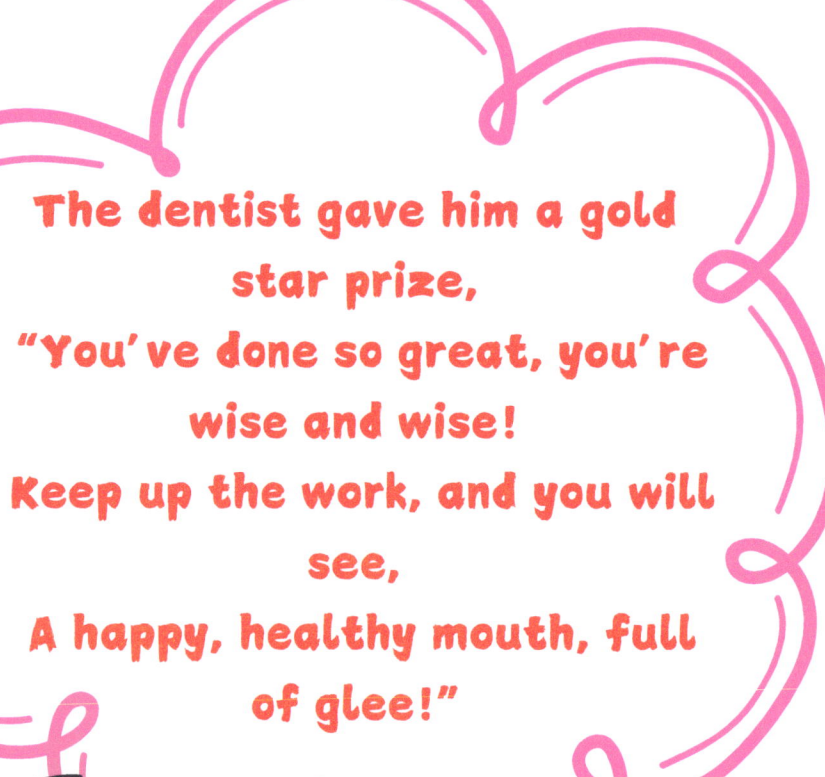

The dentist gave him a gold star prize,
"You've done so great, you're wise and wise!
Keep up the work, and you will see,
A happy, healthy mouth, full of glee!"

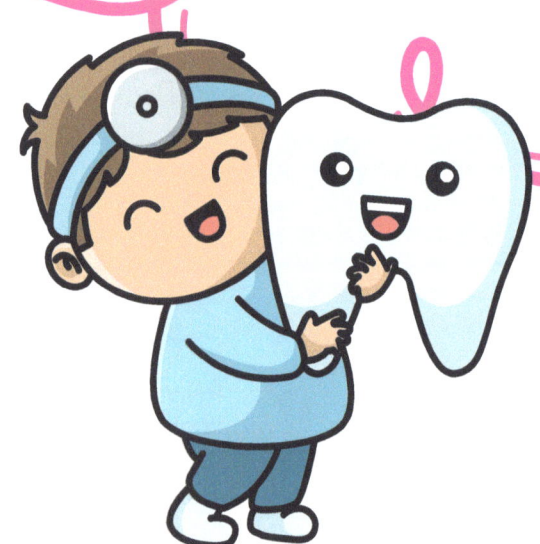

Dentist Said To Rayan

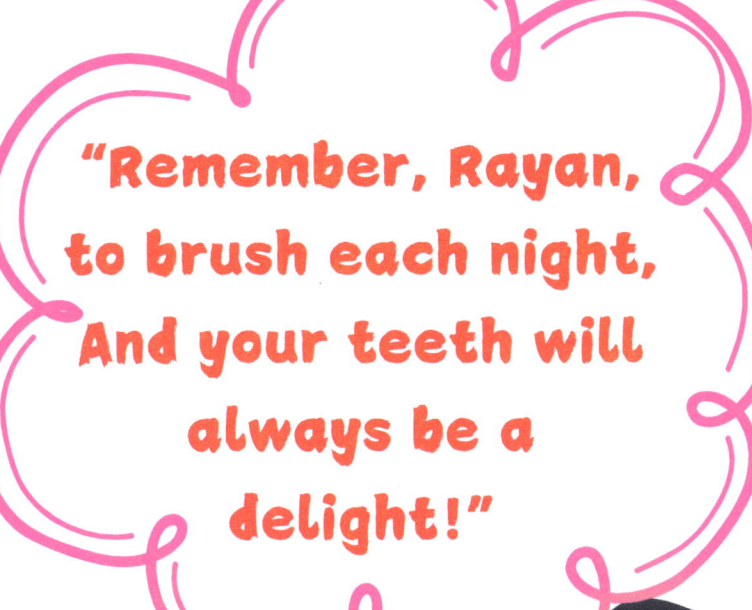

"Remember, Rayan, to brush each night, And your teeth will always be a delight!"

Dentist Said To Rayan

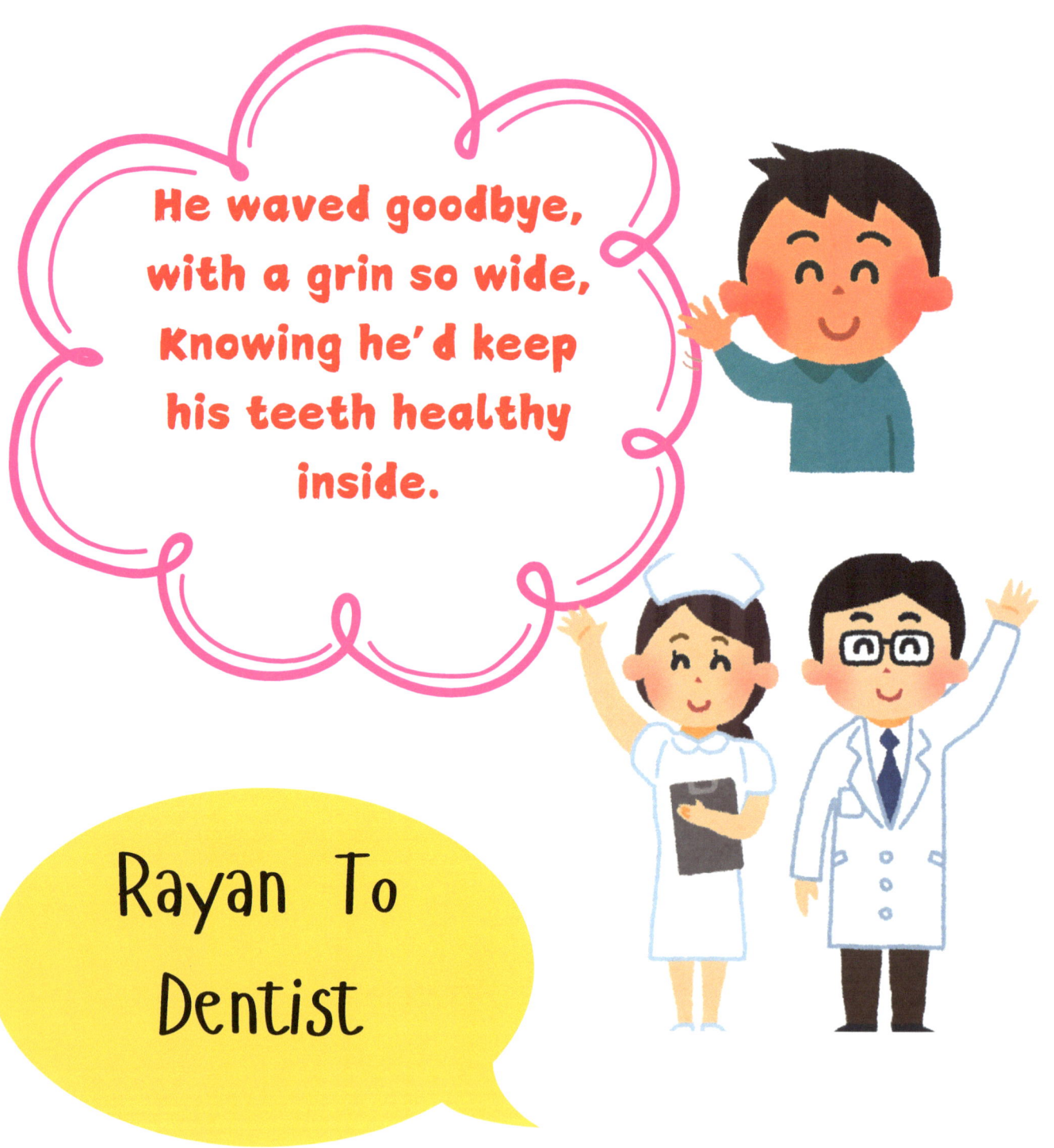

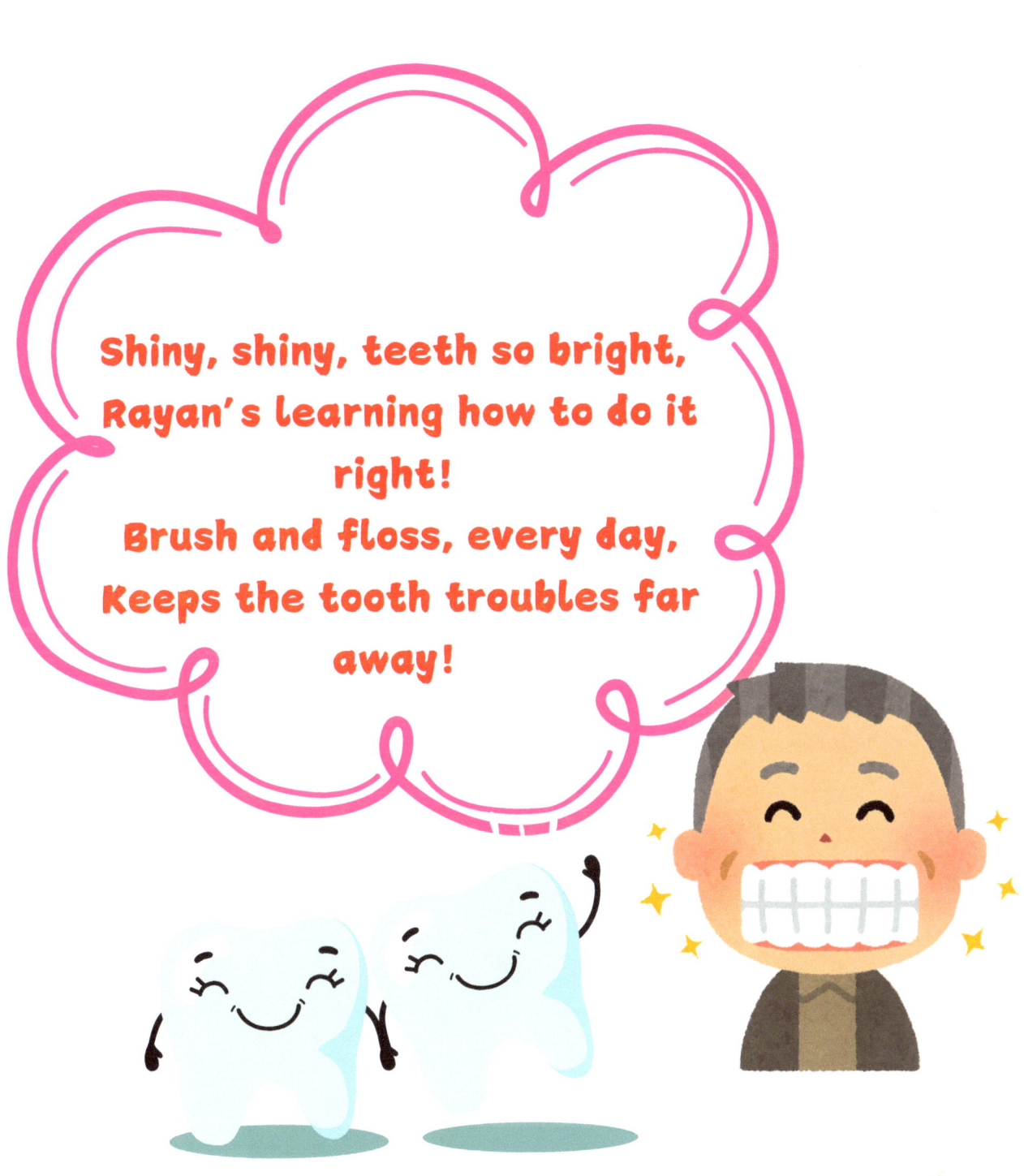

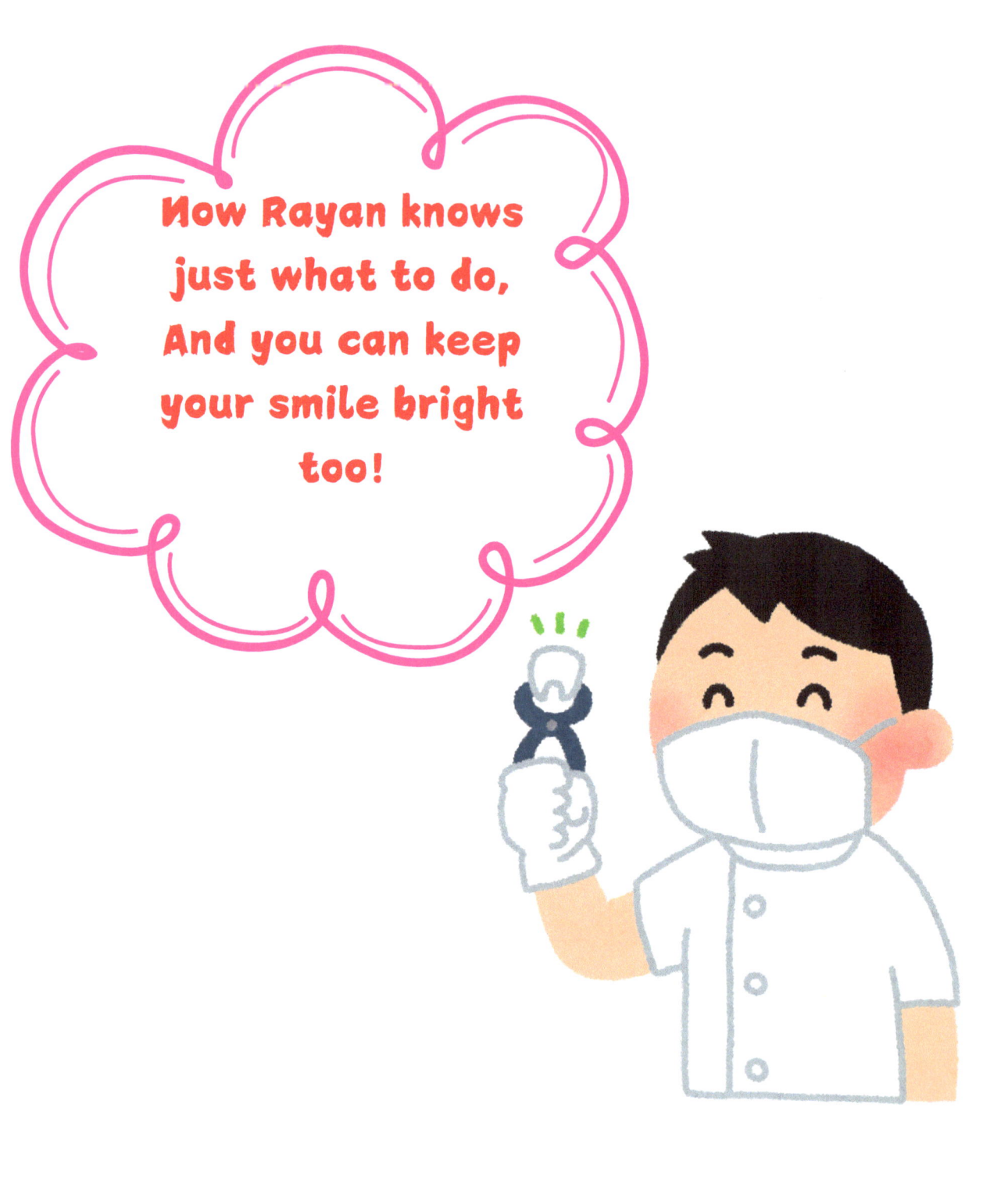

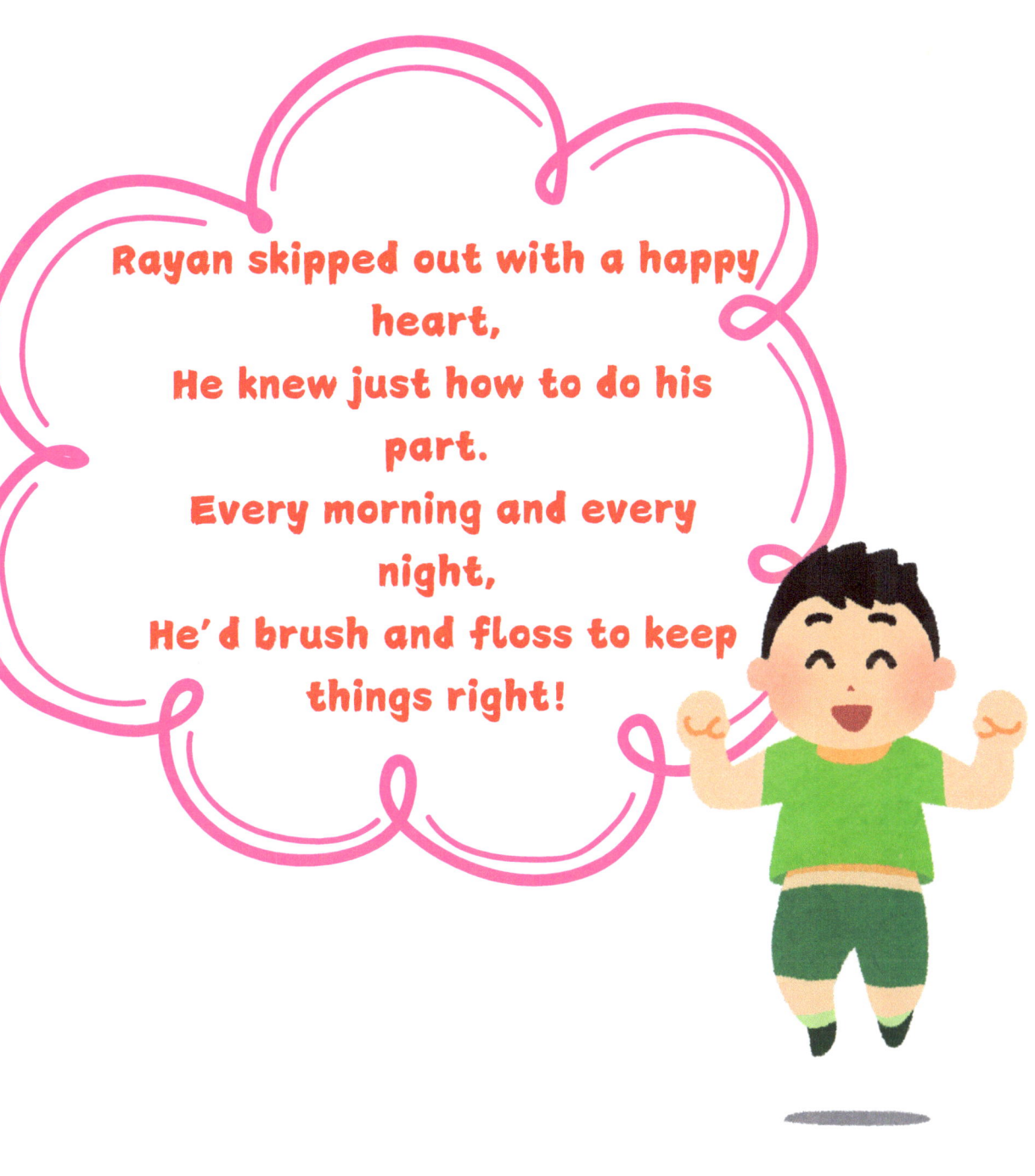

Rayan skipped out with a happy heart,
He knew just how to do his part.
Every morning and every night,
He'd brush and floss to keep things right!

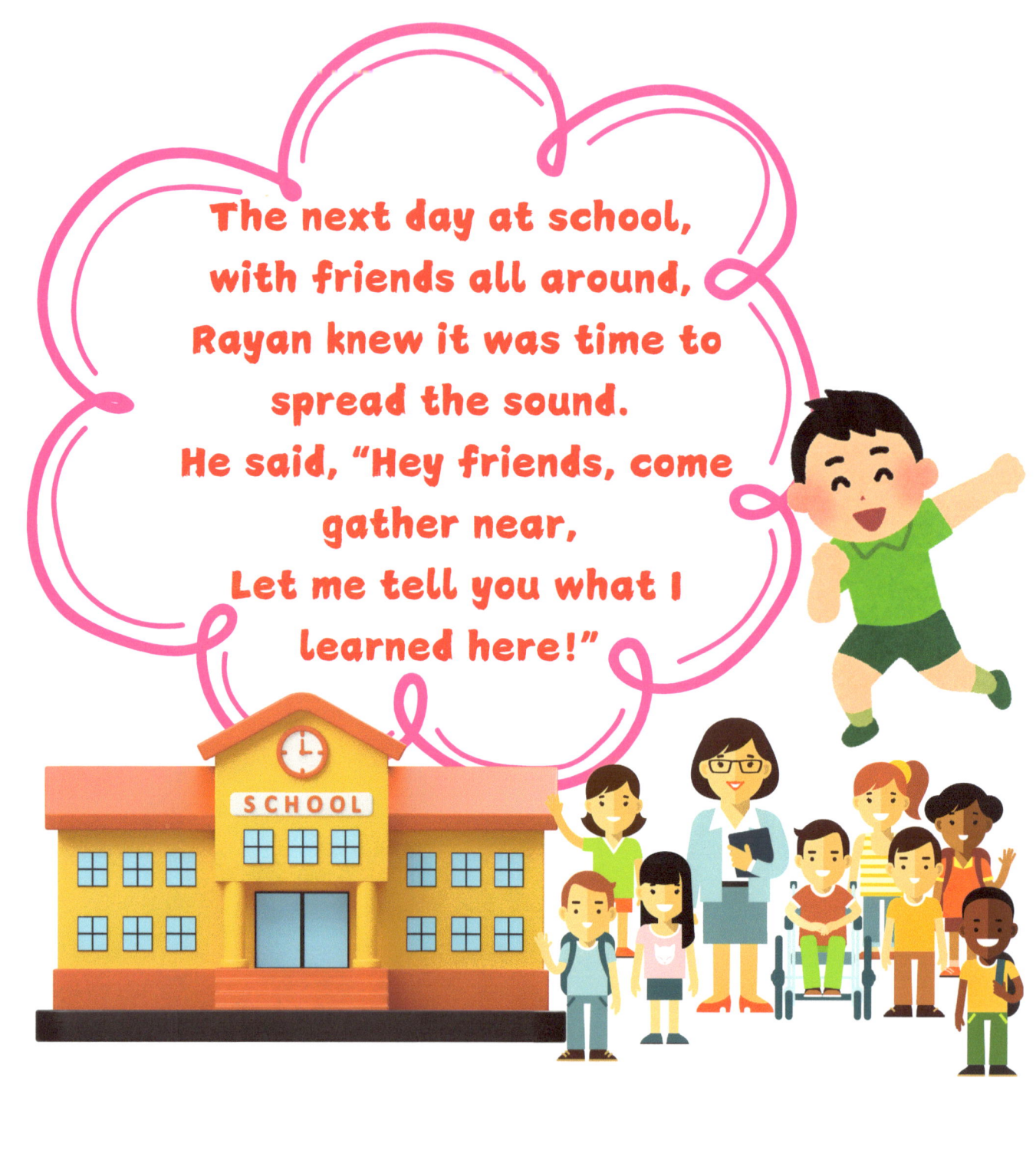

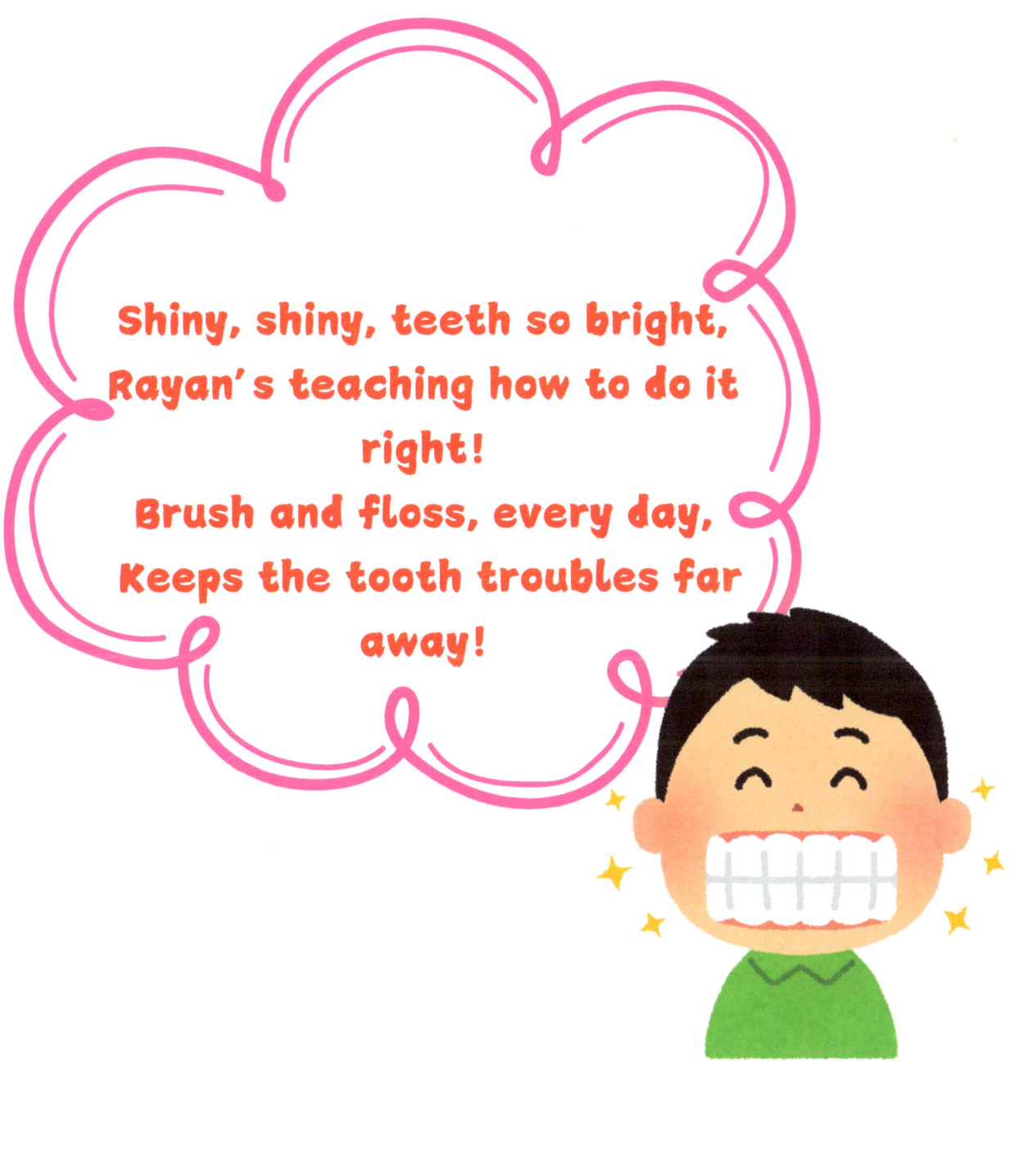

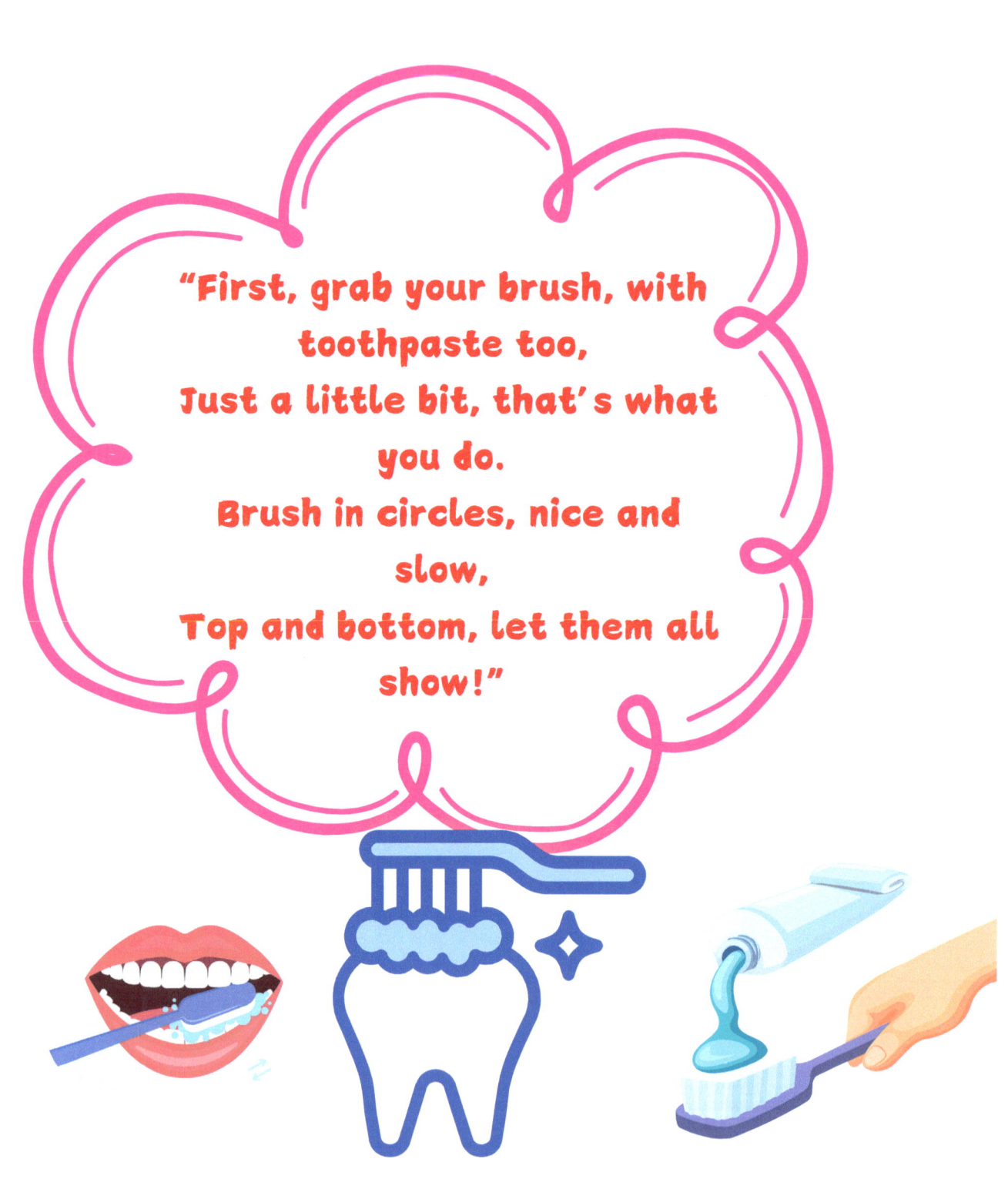

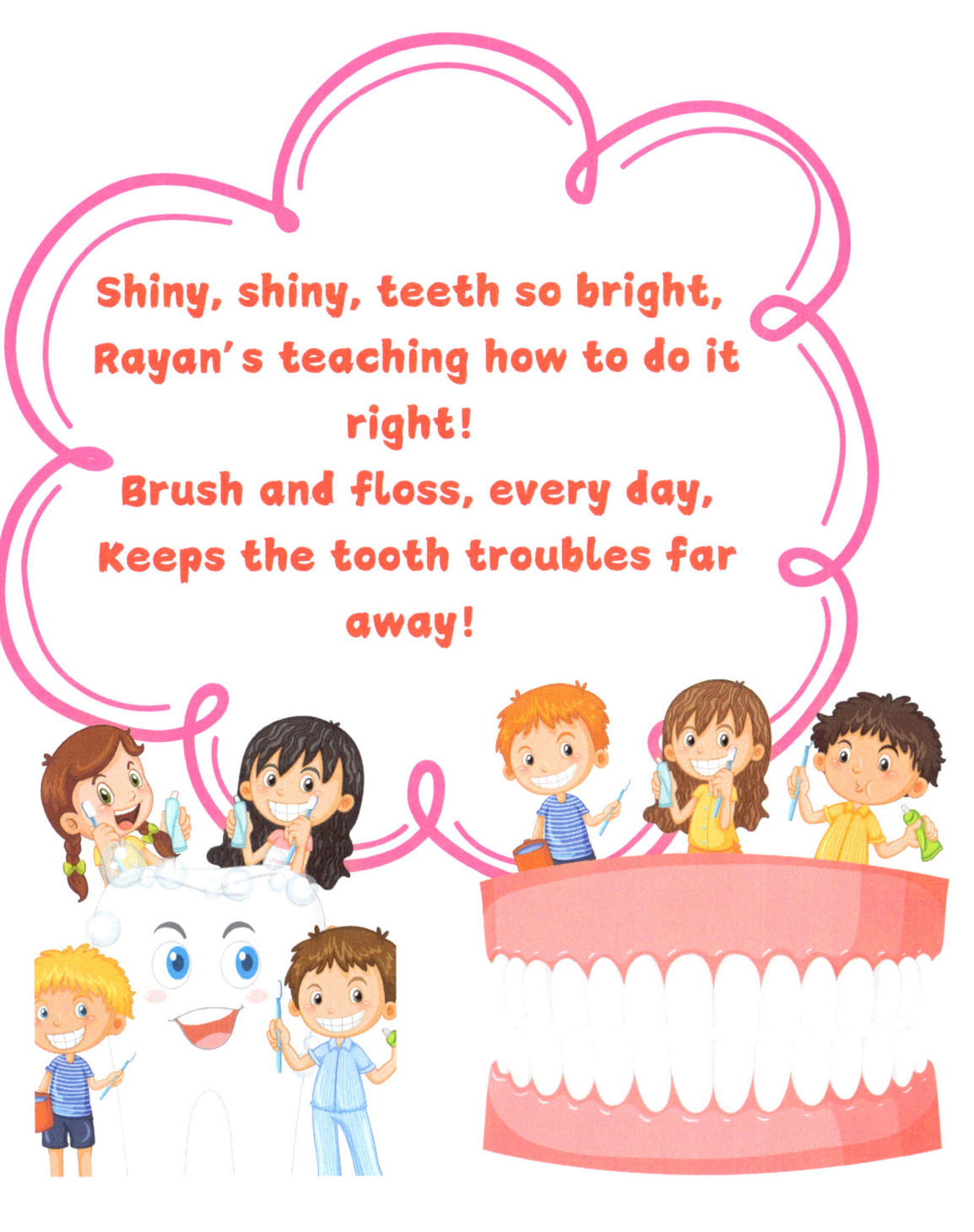

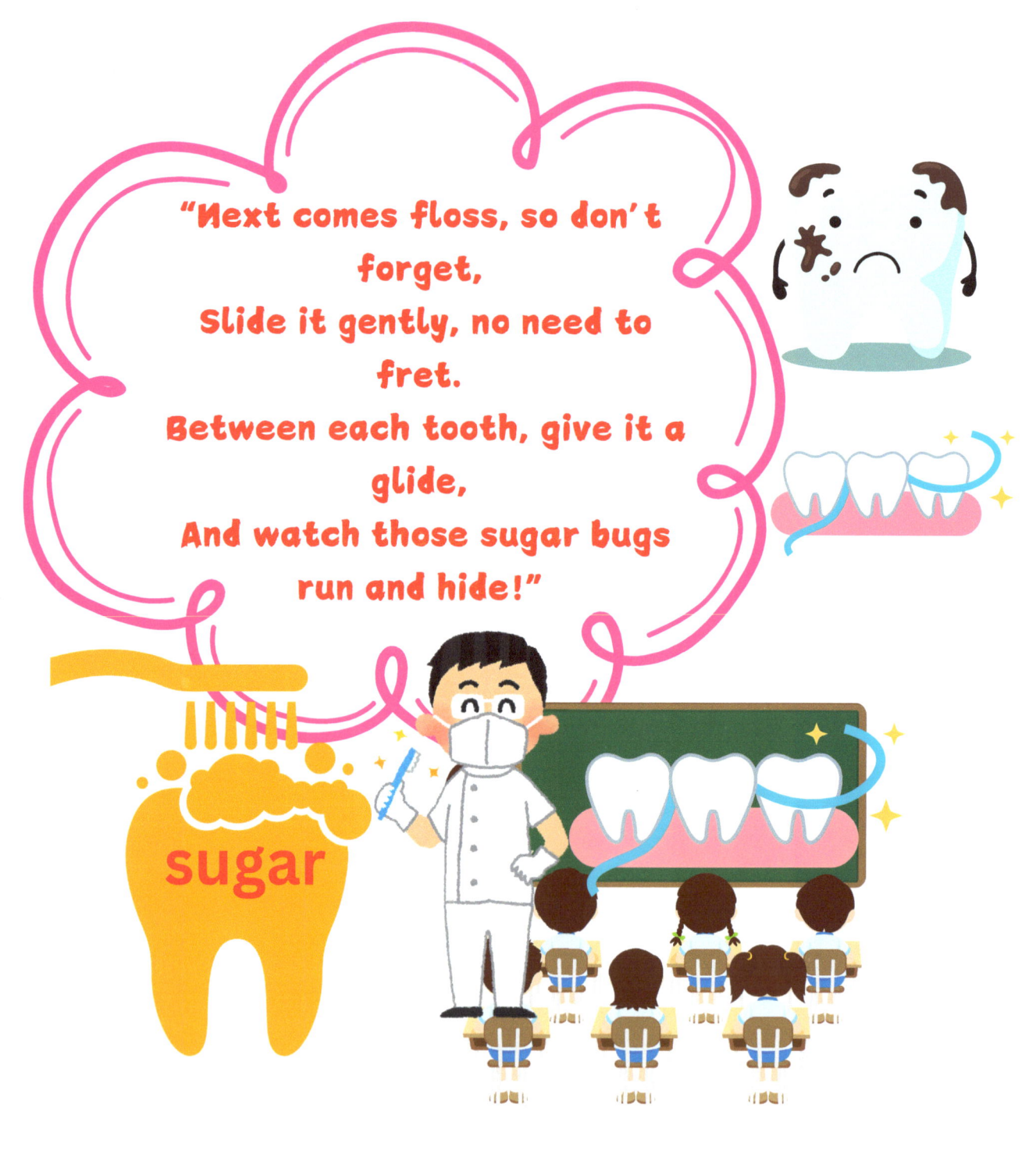

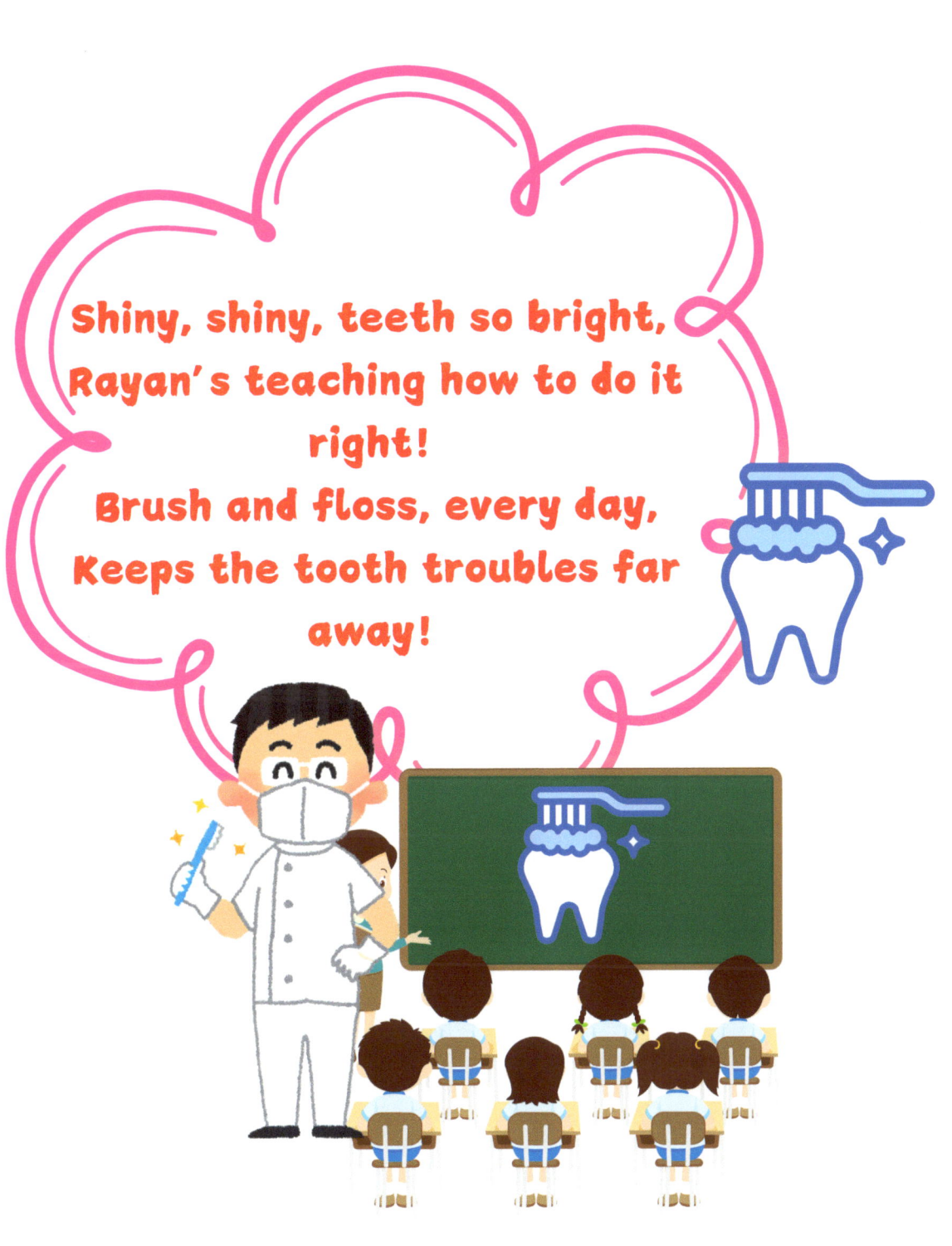

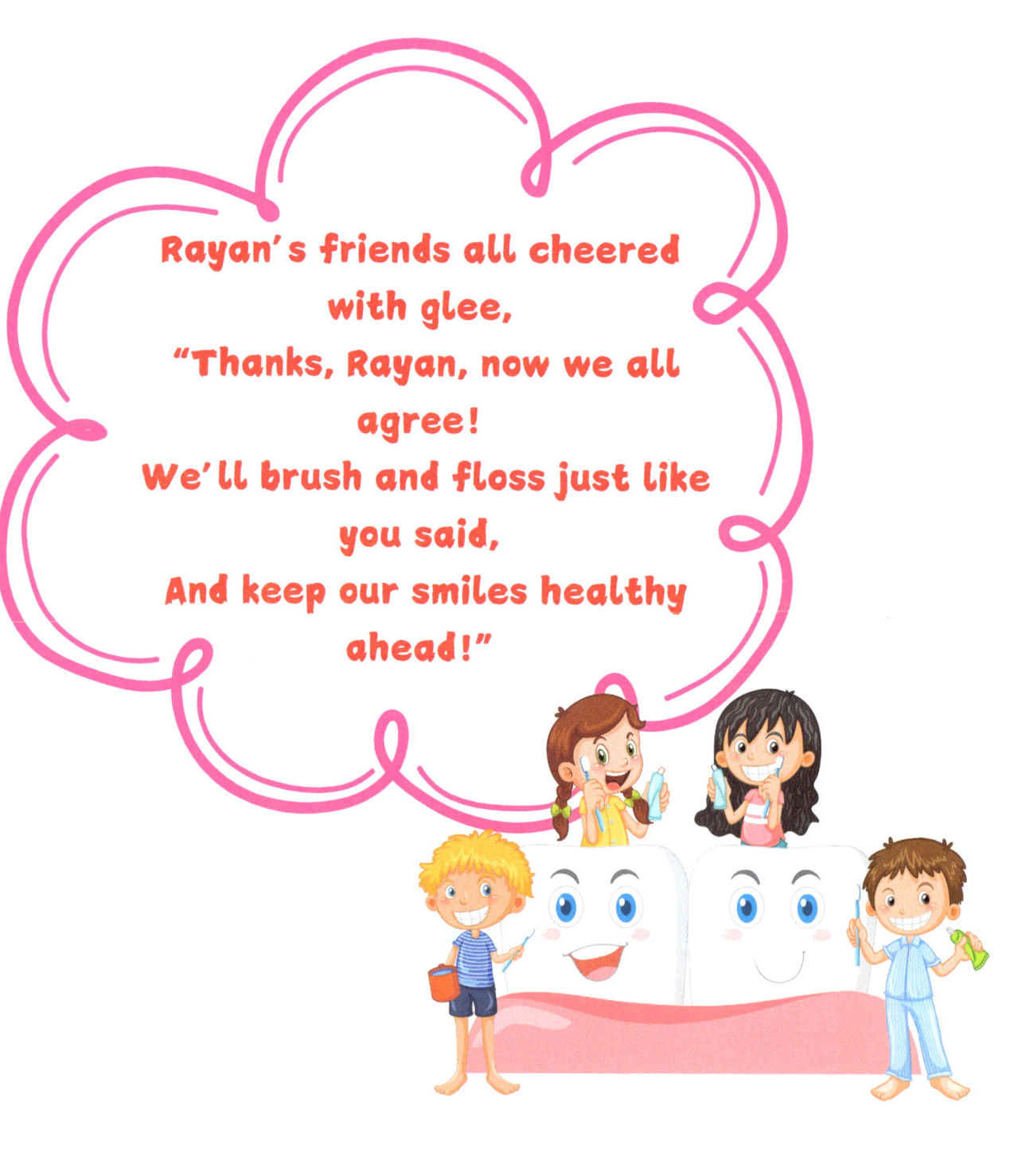

Rayan's friends all cheered with glee,
"Thanks, Rayan, now we all agree!
We'll brush and floss just like you said,
And keep our smiles healthy ahead!"

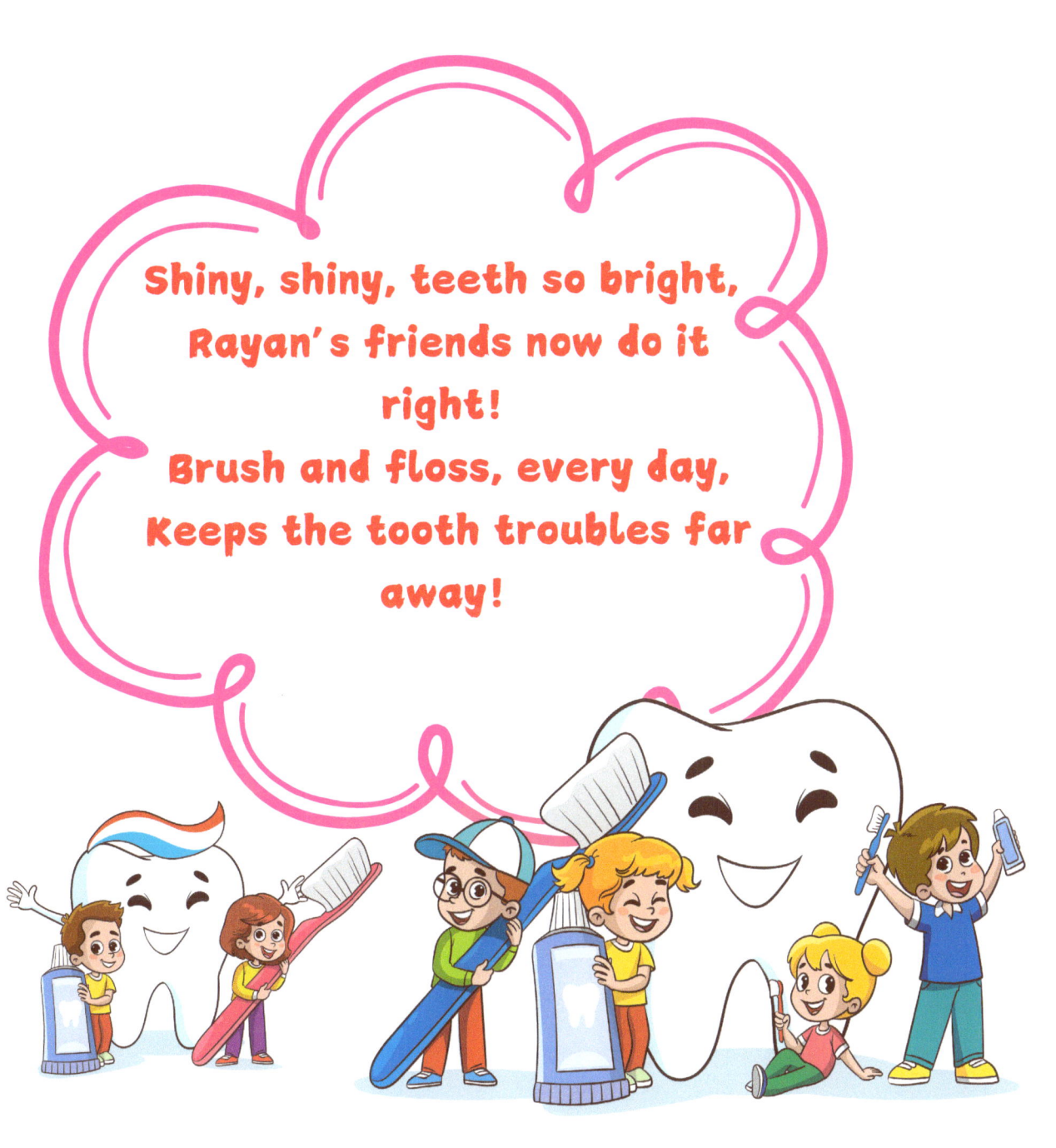

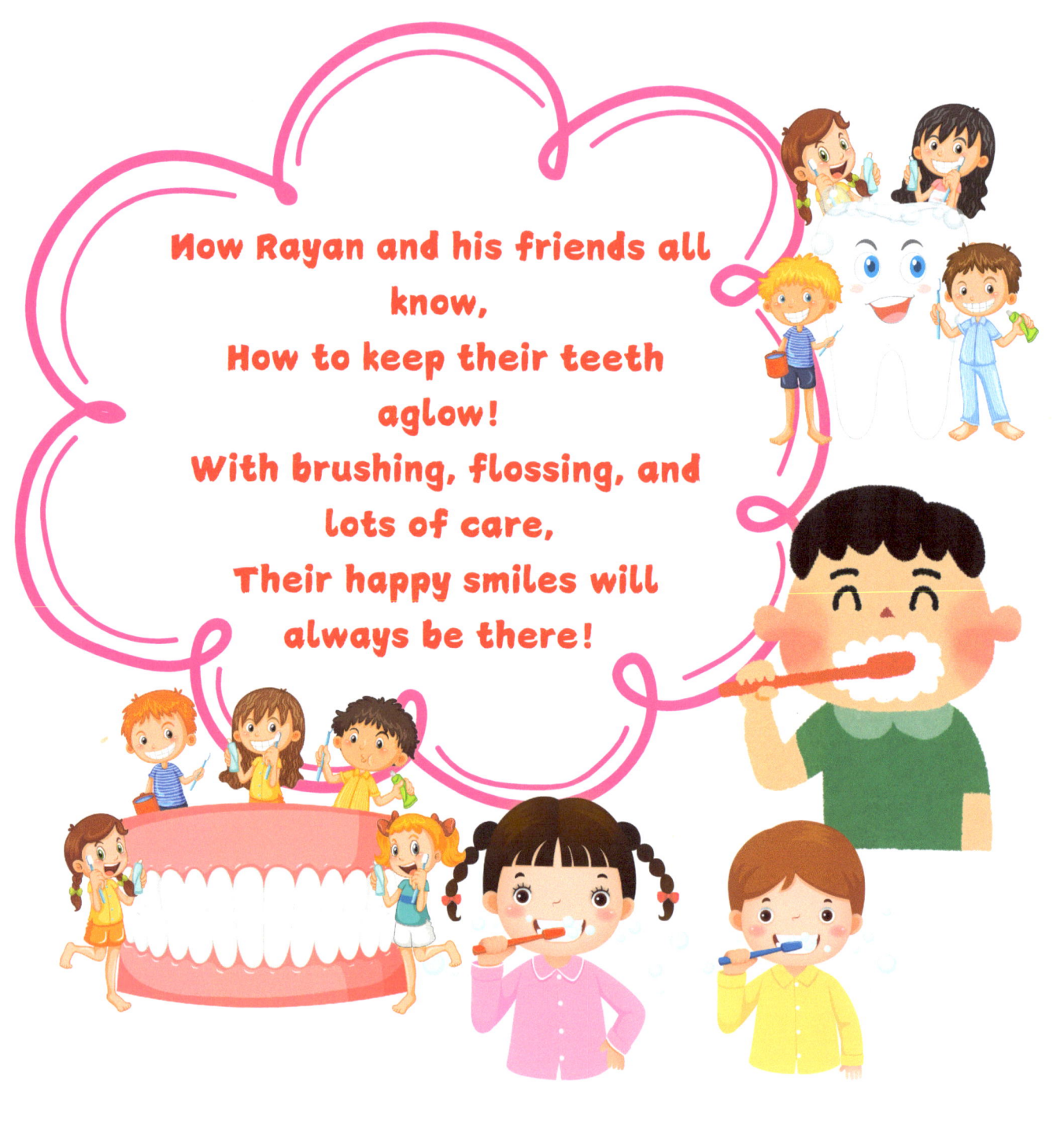

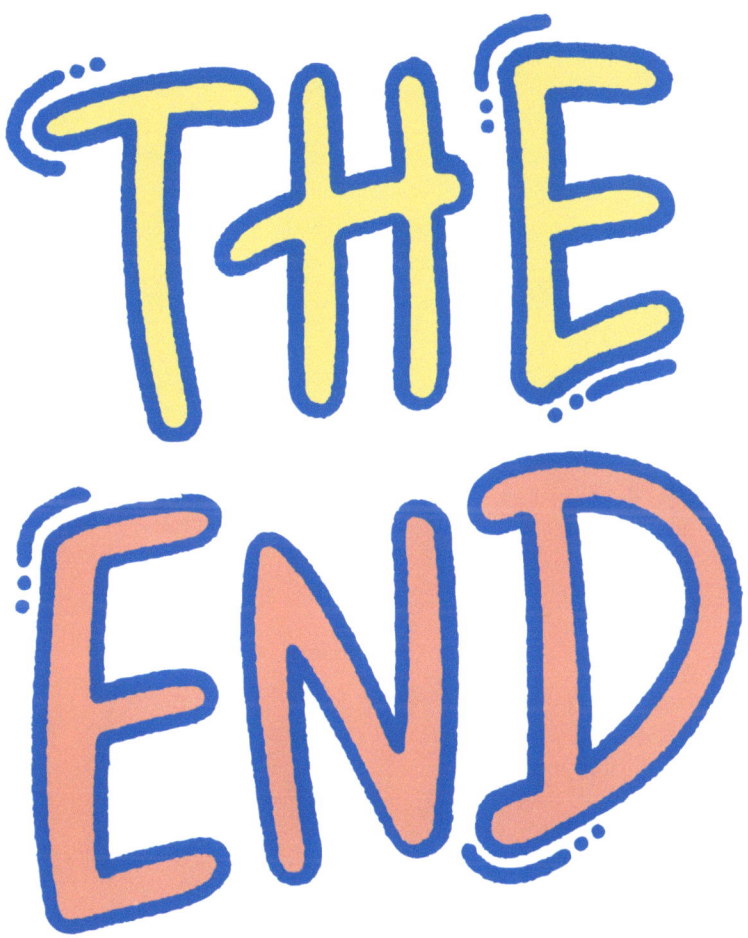

www.ingramcontent.com/pod-product-compliance
Lightning Source LLC
Chambersburg PA
CBHW040454220526
45473CB00004B/1627